AF851279

90 0514273 1

# Psychopharmacology Series 8

# Methodology of the Evaluation of Psychotropic Drugs

Edited by
O. Benkert, W. Maier, and K. Rickels

With 19 Figures

Springer-Verlag Berlin Heidelberg New York
London Paris Tokyo Hong Kong

Professor Dr. med. OTTO BENKERT

Priv.-Doz. Dr. med. WOLFGANG MAIER
Klinikum der Johannes Gutenberg-Universität Mainz,
Psychiatrische Klinik und Poliklinik, Untere Zahlbacher Straße 8,
6500 Mainz, FRG

KARL RICKELS, M.D.
University of Pennsylvania, Department of Psychiatry,
203 Piersol Building, University Hospital, 3400 Spruce Street,
Philadelphia, PA 19104-4283, USA

Vols. 1 and 2 of this series appeared under the titel „Psychopharmacology Supplementum"

ISBN 3-540-52094-5 Springer-Verlag Berlin Heidelberg New York
ISBN 0-387-52094-5 Springer-Verlag New York Berlin Heidelberg

Library of Congress Cataloging-in-Publication Data Methodology of the evaluation of psychotropic drugs / editors, O. Benkert, W. Maier, K. Rickels. p.cm. -- (Psychopharmacology series ; 8) ISBN 0-387-52094-5 (U.S. : alk. paper) 1. Psychotropic drugs--Testing. 2. Clinical trials. I. Benkert, O. II. Maier, W. (Wolfgang). III. Rickels, Karl. IV. Series. [DNLM: 1. Clinical Trials--methods. 2. Psychotropic Drugs. W1 PS773J v. 8 / QV 77 M592] RM315.M46 1990 615'.788--dc20 DNLM/DLC for Library of Congress.

This work is subject to copyright. All rights are reserved, whether the whole or part of the material is concerned, specifically the rights of translation, reprinting, re-use of illustrations, recitation, broadcasting, reproduction on microfilms or in other ways, and storage in data banks. Duplication of this publication or parts thereof is only permitted under the provisions of the German Copyright Law of September 9, 1965, in its current version, and a copyright fee must always be paid. Violations fall under the prosecution act of the German Copyright Law.

© Springer-Verlag Berlin Heidelberg 1990
Printed in Germany

The use of registered names, trademarks, etc. in this publication does not imply, even in the absence of a specific statement, that such names are exempt from the relevant protective laws and regulations and therefore free for general use.

Product Liability: The publisher can give no guarantee for information about drug dosage and application thereof contained in this book. In every individual case the respective user must check its accuracy by consulting other pharmaceutical literature.

Typesetting: International Typesetters Inc., Makati, Philippines
2125/3130(3011)-543210 – Printed on acid-free paper

# Preface

The idea of placebo-controlled drug trials and the advent of test statistics during the first part of this century were the major milestones in the establishment of a convincing methodology for demonstrating the efficacy of treatments. The first tricyclic and neuroleptic drugs were tested for their efficacy in psychiatric disorders along the lines of these methodological developments, but subsequent trials with psychotropic drugs did not adhere to these principles to the same extent because it became difficult to justify placebo-controlled trials once effective treatments had been established. Consequently, the second generation of antidepressants and neuroleptics (since the early 1960s) were mainly tested, in Europe at least, in samples of patients using trials controlled by standard treatment only, and the methodological basis of these second generation trials became fragile, as will be demonstrated by several papers in this book. This development did not provoke much discussion until recently, when scientific and administrative interest in the methodology of the evaluation of psychotropic drugs increased substantially.

A series of factors contribute to the growing interest in the standards of psychotropic drug trials:

1. The proportion of psychiatric patients resistant to treatment is growing; the efficacy of well-established forms of treatment therefore seems to be limited.
2. A series of psychotropic drugs were withdrawn from the market, mainly because they caused serious side effects. The efficacy and safety of these drugs had previously been demonstrated in drug trials, which raised the question whether the drug trials carried out were well-designed.
3. Some psychotropic drugs introduced as efficacious treatments do not meet clinicians' expectations with regard to their efficacy.
4. The number of conditions to be treated with psychopharmacological drugs is increasing. Panic and eating disorders, for example, used to be mainly treated with psychotherapy, but recent opinion increasingly considers them responsive to psychopharmacological treatment.
5. The legal and administrative regulations for the advission of psychotropic drugs are very different in different countries: in the United States, for example, the conditions are stricter than in West Germany (e.g., with respect to the need for placebo-controlled trials). The European Community will be given responsibility for licensing new drugs in Europe in 1992, making it necessary for the national administrative and legal rules in Europe to be standardized.

6. The ethical situation of psychotropic drug trials is becoming more and more complicated. It becomes harder to justify new drug trials the more effective treatments already exist. Additional ethical criteria to be applied differ according to nation.
7. The number of patients available for drug trials is decreasing for a variety of reasons, including a higher refutation rate and the increased number of inpatients refractory to standard outpatient treatment. Other limitations concerning treatment are equally relevant in current drug trials (e.g., long duration of pretreatment, need for concomitant treatment).
8. Methodological problems have been recognized as inherent in the current state of psychotropic drug trials, but simple solutions to these problems are not available.
9. The methodology of testing the efficacy of some kinds of psychotropic drugs (e.g., nootropics – cognition-enhancing drugs) is extremely controversial.

The administration of a drug in the treatment of patients requires the clinical efficacy and safety of the drug to have been demonstrated prior to use. It is evident that the process of testing drug efficacy should be standardized for each category of drugs (antidepressants, anxiolytics, neuroleptics, hypnotics, nootropics), but methodological standards for testing the therapeutic efficacy of a drug have changed substantially since the first tricyclic antidepressant and neuroleptic drugs were introduced. Therefore, the existence of criteria for establishing efficacy unique to each category of psychotropic drugs is open to discussion. In this book, the editors have attempted to describe the present state of the art and to indicate unsolved and controversial problems, and have proposed solutions for the evaluation of psychotropic drugs.

Unfortunately, any overview on problems and possible solutions is not perfect. Drug trials in clinical settings (late phase II or phase III) are the focus of all contributions; it was not intended to discuss preclinical trials. The first four chapters on antidepressants, anxiolytics, neuroleptics, hypnotics, and nootropics are devoted to the current standard of drug evaluation for each of these categories of drugs, with particular regard to the current status in terms of selection criteria, length of drug trials, measures of efficacy, and the need for placebo-controlled trials. The drugs able to serve as active treatment controls are identified and recommendations to overcome the methodological flaws of the current drug evaluation studies are given. These presentations of the current state of the evaluation of psychotropic drugs are not intended to be exhaustive; the four chapters discuss mainly controversial issues of current interest. A series of conditions currently being tested for their response to psychotropic drugs are not included in these overviews (e.g., obsessive-compulsive disorder, eating disorder, somatization disorders). The chapter by Crook on the evaluation of nootropic drugs includes a proposal for the measurement of efficacy in cognition enhancing Drugs. Levine subsequently discusses the current strategies in the ascertainment of side effects in clinical trials.

The chapter by Paykel on placebo-controlled drug studies in depression demonstrates the feasibility of placebo use, defines the need for it, and identifies indicators for these kinds of studies. The chapter on the design of drug trials by Helmchen focuses on the ethical implications involved and proposes guidelines for the selection of inclusion and exclusion criteria and for determining the duration and conduct of treatment in controlled trials.

Biostatistical issues which should be taken into consideration in designing and evaluating drug trials are discussed in a chapter by Lavori, which focuses on requirements for sample size and for handling drop outs in evaluating drug trials.

The psychopathological aspects of drug trials relevant to the measurement of efficacy and to the definition of selection criteria are the topic of four chapters. Two of them are dedicated to the measurement of drug effects as defined by psychopathological items (Maier, Bech), one discusses diagnosis as selection criteria of drug trials (Buller), and the chapter by Benkert presents new conceptual developments in classifying psychiatric patients according to their response to treatment and the consequences of these developments for the identification of drug-responsive patients.

The concluding chapter by Müller-Oerlinghausen provides an overview of the current status of guidelines proposed by various international committees. The relevance and justification of such guidelines remains an unsolved issue, however, which cannot be discussed extensively in this monograph.

The majority of the chapters of this book were based on presentations given in a symposium on the "Methodology of the Evaluation of Psychotropic Drugs" on the occasion of the congress of the Collegium Internationale Neuropsychopharmacologicum (CINP), August 1988 in Munich.

The editors hope that this book will be of interest to clinicians and psychopharmacologists interested in familiarizing themselves with the current state of the art in the methodology developed to test the efficacy of psychotropic drugs.

Mainz and Philadelphia, Spring 1990

O. Benkert, W. Maier, and K. Rickels

# Contents

# List of Contributors

You will find the addresses at the beginning of the respective contribution.

# State of the Art in Drug Trials

# Evaluating Antidepressants and Anxiolytics

K. RICKELS[1]

## 1 Introduction

During recent years, many experimental compounds have entered the clinical research arena. The hope has been to find effective anxiolytics and antidepressants, with clinical efficacy at least as great as such standards as diazepam for anxiety and imipramine or amitriptyline for depression, but at the same time with a milder adverse event profile. For anxiolytics, this would translate primarily into producing less sedation and no dependency-producing properties, and for antidepressants primarily an absence or reduction of anticholinergic properties, excessive sedation, orthostatic hypertension, and cardiac toxicity.

As diagnostic criteria have become more atheoretical and more operationally definable (DSM-III-R, American Psychiatric Association 1987); research patients can be described more clearly and, consequently, results across research groups and even across national boundaries are more comparable.

A number of excellent guidelines have been published to guide researchers in developing clinical research protocols. Most, however, antedate the introduction of the DSM-III-R. These guidelines have been published in attempts to resolve methodological problems and inconsistencies in clinical trials. Among these guidelines are the "*General Consideration of the Clinical Evaluation of Drugs*" (FDA 1977), as well as the "*Guidelines for the Clinical Evaluation of Psychotropic Drugs, Antidepressant and Anti-anxiety Drugs*" (FDA 1978). The latter guidelines also carefully discuss appropriate approaches to be used when a new agent is given to humans for the first time, i.e., in phase 1 of drug development. Similar guidelines, with only minor modifications, have been published by the World Health Organization (Sartorius et al. 1988) and by Wittenborn (1977). Two publications of particular relevance to the topic at hand are *Principles and Problems of Establishing the Efficacy of Psychotropic Agents,* edited by Levine et al. and published in 1971; and *Coordinating Clinical Trials in Psychopharmacology: Planning, Documentation, and Analysis,* edited by Levine and published in 1979. While these publications are many years old already, they are, with the exception of diagnostic definitions, as new as if they had been written recently.

---

* The preparation of this paper was supported in part by USPHS Research Grant MH08957.

[1] Psychopharmacology Research and Treatment Unit, Department of Psychiatry, University of Pennsylvania, Philadelphia, PA 19104, USA

Methodology of the Evaluation of Psychotropic Drugs
Editors: O. Benkert, W. Maier, and K. Rickels
(Psychopharmacology Series 8)
© Springer-Verlag Berlin Heidelberg 1990

The ACNP's publication *Psychopharmacology: The Third Generation of Progress* also offers a section dealing with methodology of clinical trials (Overall 1987; Levine and Ban 1987; Goldberg 1987; Overall and Rhoades 1987).

Rather than repeating everything already said in some or all of the publications mentioned, as well as in many others, this chapter will focus on what I hold to be some of the more important aspects of clinical trial methodology. These considerations are based on more than 25 years of hands-on experience in the field of clinical drug evaluations, much of it continuously supported by the National Institute of Mental Health (NIMH). I have also been intimately involved in the development of the early FDA as well as international guidelines. Thus, it is hoped that the reader will derive benefits from this chapter, as a help in the design, conduct, or sponsoring of clinical trials in anxiety and depression.

In another chapter, ethical issues involved in conducting drug trials in humans are extensively discussed. I would be remiss, however, not to mention that no clinical trial should be conducted that has not previously been reviewed by a properly constituted Institutional Review Board, and before the patient has given his or her written voluntary informed consent to participate in the proposed "experimental" drug trial.

## 2 Study Sample

The subjects of a given study have to be clearly described according to several parameters (Table 1). These should include a present DSM-III-R, ICD 9CM (American Psychiatric Association 1987) diagnosis, or Research Diagnostic Criteria (RDC) (Spitzer et al. 1978), as well as several operational definitions beyond those demanded for a DSM-III-R diagnosis (e.g., the presence of a certain score on an anxiety or depression intake checklist) (FDA 1978). The *patient sample* should also be described in terms of several rating scale cutoff points necessary for entering the trial, as, for example, a cutoff score of 18 to 20 on the Hamilton Anxiety Scale (Hamilton 1959), or Hamilton Depression 17 or 21-item scale (Hamilton 1960), and a cutoff score of 9 on the Covi anxiety (Lipman and Covi 1976) or Raskin depression (Raskin et al. 1970) screen, with the Covi score being higher than the Raskin score for anxiety studies, the Raskin being higher than the Covi score for depression studies. In both anxiety and depression studies, the CGI global psychopathology (Guy 1976) score should be at least 4 on a scale from 1 to 7, and on the Hopkins Symptom Checklist (Derogatis et al. 1974), patients should be at least 2 standard deviations above normal scores in either anxiety or depression. For panic disorder, the most important criterion is the number of major panic attacks per week, and the degree of phobic avoidance present (Ballenger et al. 1988).

Some of the most important DSM-III-R *diagnostic criteria* are given in Table 2. They include generalized anxiety disorder (GAD), panic disorder (PD), anxiety not otherwise specified (NOS), adjustment disorder, as well as various phobic and obsessive-compulsive disorders. The major diagnostic criteria for depression are major depressive disorder (MDD), and bipolar disorder, depressed type.

**Table 1.** Study sample

*Diagnosis*

- DSM-III-R, ICD9-CM
- Operational definition: FDA guidelines, European guidelines, St. Louis Research Diagnostic Criteria (RDC)
- Rating scale cutoff points
  - Hamilton Anxiety or Depression Rating Scale
  - Covi-Raskin Scales
  - CGI – Global Psychopathology Scale
  - Hopkins Symptom Checklist (HSCL) – anxiety or depression factor
  - Number of major panic attacks
  - Global assessment of phobic avoidance
- Structured interviews: SADS-L, SCID

*Psychiatric/medical history*

- Demographics
- Illness history
- Duration of present episode
- Previous psychiatric episodes
- Previous psychiatric treatment with/without medication
- Precipitating events
- Family/occupational/social functioning
- Coffee/alcohol intake
- Intercurrent medical illnesses and treatments
- Family history of psychiatric illness

*Inclusion and exclusion criteria*

- Clearly specified for each study

**Table 2.** Some DSM-III-R diagnoses

| | |
|---|---|
| *Anxiety* | |
| 300.02 | Generalized anxiety disorder (GAD), with or without depression |
| 300.00 | Anxiety disorder not otherwise specified (NOS) |
| 300.01 | Panic disorder (PD), without agoraphobia |
| 300.21 | Panic disorder (PD), with agoraphobia |
| 300.23 | Social phobia |
| 300.30 | Obsessive-compulsive disorder |
| 309.24 | Adjustment disorder with anxious mood |
| *Depression* | |
| 296.2 | Major depressive disorder (MDD), single episode |
| 296.3 | Major depressive disorder (MDD), recurrent episode |
| 296.5 | Bipolar disorder, depressed |
| 300.4 | Dysthymia (depressive neurosis), primary or secondary |
| 309.00 | Adjustment disorder with depressed mood |

Most researchers quite correctly exclude adjustment disorders and dysthymia as primary diagnostic research criteria. Yet many GAD patients probably also fulfill the secondary diagnostic criterion for dysthymia. The problem with dysthymia is that it combines chronicity with minor depressive symptomatology. Thus, most physicians who make a GAD diagnosis, would probably diagnose such patients as suffering from GAD with secondary depressive features rather than using the DSM-III-R diagnostic criteria of dysthymia as a secondary diagnosis.

For depression, it is also important to divide patients into endogenous or nonendogenous patients (Spitzer et al. 1978), or into patients suffering from melancholia or not (American Psychiatric Association 1987). It is important to divide depressed patients into endogenous and nonendogenous subtypes, because patients diagnosed as nonendogenous have a higher placebo response rate than endogenously depressed patients, frequently negating any drug-placebo differences for this large depression subgroup (Table 3).

At all times, diagnoses must be clearly defined, and investigators should use short, well-defined, cookbook-type, structured diagnostic checklists based on DSM-III-R or RDC criteria to diagnose their patients.

The use of large-scale *structured interviews* lasting about 1 h, such as the Schedule for Affective Disorder and Schizophrenia, Lifetime version (SADS-L) (Endicott and Spitzer 1978), or the Structured Clinical Interview for DSM-III (SCID) (Spitzer and Williams 1983), is not necessary in most clinical trials. Such interviews may occasionally be used, however, when lower-level health professionals are given the task of diagnosing patients. In general, however, our research group found that the structured interview does not replace a well-trained research physician who, with the help of a short, one- to three-page structured checklist, based on the DSM-III-R criteria, will make an appropriate diagnosis.

Table 4 compares a patient's diagnostic assessment made by a research-trained family physician using a DSM-III checklist, and an independent diagnosis made by a Ph.D. psychologist based on a SADS-L interview (unpublished data). Using the Kappa value as a measure of agreement, one clearly sees that diagnoses made by both methods are in almost full agreement. A full-sized structured interview would therefore not have been necessary in this instance.

It should be stressed, however, that our raters have been intensively trained (Rickels et al. 1977) and retrained, and regularly participate in videotaped ratings

**Table 3.** Improved depressed patients at treatment endpoint ($\geq$ 50% decrease in Hamilton Depression Scale) (in percent)

| | Endogenous | Reactive | $X^2$ | $P$ |
|---|---|---|---|---|
| Tricyclic (lofepramine) ($n$ = 89) | 60 | 62 | 0.03 | n.s. |
| Placebo ($n$ = 93) | 27 | 56 | 7.72 | $P < .01$ |

**Table 4.** Concordance between trial physician's diagnosis and SADS-L diagnosis

| | Trial physician | |
|---|---|---|
| | Predominantly anxious | Predominantly depressed |
| SADS-L | | |
| Predominantly anxious | 85 | 4 |
| Predominantly depressed | 6 | 74 |
| kappa = 0.88 | | |

or in joint ratings with another rater of individual patients. Such highly trained individuals will indeed produce a high correlation with a structured interview, but such high correlation could certainly not be expected for a physician who conducts clinical research for the first time or only rarely, and at the most participates in a 1-day training session conducted by the pharmaceutical sponsor of his study.

In my opinion, some of the main roles of structured interviews are to:

1. Facilitate the training of physicians, raters, and other mental health professionals
2. Assure quality control by examining subgroups of a larger study population with such an interview
3. Assure a correct diagnosis if persons other than the physician are assigned the task of diagnosing psychiatric patients.

If one finds, for example, deviations between a structured interview and the physician's independently made diagnosis, one may institute additional training sessions, search for reasons for such discrepancies, or possibly replace such physician or researcher in the present as well as future studies.

Several *prestudy variables* that should be obtained in any trial are shown in Table 1. They are collected for two main reasons: to allow for an appropriate study replication by other investigators, and to permit the search for possible predictors of treatment response (Rickels 1968). Even such information as caffeine intake may provide important data, as excessive caffeine intake may well lead to increased anxiety and sleeplessness, and if suddenly stopped, even to withdrawal reactions which may mistakenly be associated by both patient and physician with the treatment medication. Caffeine use, as well as smoking, may also counteract drug-induced sedative side effects (Downing and Rickels 1981).

*Inclusion and exclusion* criteria must be expressly specified for a given study, and should include, particularly in early phase 2 research, an exclusion of women of childbearing potential. This limitation may be lifted as soon as some preliminary evidence of efficacy has been found, and as soon as all teratogenic animal studies have proved to be satisfactory.

In all discussed trials, one should ensure that a woman does not become pregnant during the course of the trial, that she uses medically accepted birth control methods, and that a pregnancy test is negative. Having a good knowledge of one's patients and accepting into a study only patients whom the physician feels sure are conscientious and who according to their past history demonstrate an ability to prevent pregnancy, will help assure that a pregnancy is avoided during a drug trial. The exclusion of women of childbearing potential from drug studies severely hinders the swift execution of clinical studies and also eliminates a large subgroup of the population who will eventually be the main user of anxiolytics and antidepressants.

Inclusion and exclusion criteria should also discuss allowed and disallowed concurrent nonpsychiatric illnesses and medications, as well as possibly allowable psychiatric medications such as chloral hydrate for sleep.

It is probably fair to say that the fewer patients have been tested with an experimental agent, the more rigorous one has to be in defining exclusion and inclusion criteria and the more frequent laboratory and EKG assessments should be made. On the other hand, once the drug has reached the phase 3 development program, one should refrain from using study populations so "pure" that once the drug is approved, hardly any patient resembles the study patients on whose response the drug approval is based.

## 3 Setting

The setting in which the research is conducted must be well described. The same is true for the amount and quality of physician-patient interaction occurring during the study (Table 5). Such interaction may well influence placebo and drug response rates (Rickels 1968). For example, physicians who, while conducting a drug trial also offer the same patients intensive group therapy experience, should state so clearly, as the amount of nondrug intervention may differ from study to study and from setting to setting, and thus may contribute significantly to observed setting x treatment interactions.

All investigators must be clinically well trained and familiar with the diagnostic patient group to be studied. Investigators must also be well trained in research methodology and able to make a correct diagnosis and to assess correctly the intensity of illness and treatment outcome. Physician and patient rater training should be ongoing, i.e., be conducted at regular intervals and include frequent video and live patient interview sessions, didactic training, and intensive protocol review and discussions (Rickels et al. 1977).

In order to assure full protocol compliance, highest research quality, and rater stability in family practice, our group has developed a procedure whereby our staff of trained raters (Ph.D.'s, M.S.W.'s, or M.D.'s) goes to the private office of our family physicians and helps them to conduct the research in their offices, including the rating of research patients and the supervision of research assistants. Private family physicians simply do not have the time to conduct research

**Table 5.** Setting – Investigators

*Setting:*

- Psychiatric clinic
- Psychiatric practice
- Symptomatic volunteers
- Family practice
- Inpatients, outpatients

*Physician/rater:*

- Experienced in clinical research
- Frequent training sessions:
  Video and live patient interviews
  Didactic training
  Intensive protocol review and discussion
- Frequent monitoring
- One investigators meeting of all investigators, usually run by sponsor prior to study beginning, not needed for some experts and too little for most physicians and raters

*Physician/patient interaction:*

- Time spent during interview
- Record of any structured nondrug therapy such as group or individual psychotherapy

interviews, and complete the myriad of research forms demanded today. Clinical research has simply become too time-consuming for a busy practice. In addition, centrally trained raters, rating patients in several family practices, introduce a measure of stability in the clinical ratings of anxious or depressed patients in the family practice setting.

Our group found it important that a one- or two-page short protocol be attached to each research patient's folder, so that the physician or rater can always refresh himself about all inclusion and exclusion criteria as well as dosage schedule relevant for the drug trial, without having to read through a lengthy protocol, amended four or five times by which time it is almost incomprehensible. Physicians who participate in clinical research also should be frequently monitored, either by the principal academic research group, the sponsor, or both.

For the evaluation of anxiolytics for the treatment of GAD and PD, family practice patients seem to represent a particularly appropriate population to be studied, but only if the family physicians, or their raters, have been adequately trained as already mentioned. Without adequate training (a 1- or 2-day prestudy meeting arranged by the sponsor does not represent adequate training), such clinical research cannot be conducted in family practice. For the evaluation of antidepressants, psychiatric research clinics and private psychiatric practices are the preferred treatment settings, followed closely by the family practice setting and only lastly by symptomatic volunteer clinics, clinics that presently are almost exclusively used in clinical research in the U.S.

## 4 Assessments

Table 6 mentions the more frequently used physician and patient rating scales for *efficacy assessment.* In addition, analogue scales (Aitken 1969) are useful to assess frequent mood changes. One example would be to assess daily mood at home during the first week of treatment if one suspects an early drug response. In any anxiety study, and until better scales become available, the Hamilton Anxiety Scale (Hamilton 1959) and the CGI global ratings of psychopathology and of

**Table 6.** Assessments

*Efficacy:*

*Physician/rater*

- Hamilton Anxiety Scale
- Hamilton Depression Scale
- Montgomery-Asberg Depression Scale
- CGI/global psychopathology
- Scale to assess panic attacks and phobic avoidance behavior
- Mood Analogue Scales
- Global improvement
- Other

*Patient*

- Hopkins Symptom Checklist (HSCL)
- Profile of Mood Scale (POMS)
- Zung Anxiety Scale
- Zung Depression Scale
- von Zerssen Beschwerdeliste
- Global Improvement
- Quality of Life Assessments
- Other

*Adverse events*

- Global, indirect
- Specific inquiry (TESS, SAFTEE)
- Rebound anxiety/depression
- Prolonged withdrawal
- Return of original symptoms

*Miscellaneous*

- Concurrent illness and medication
- External events
- Drug plasma determinations
- Psychomotor/cognitive/memory assessments
- Study drug-taking record/pill counts
- Vital signs, laboratory tests, EKG, physical examination

*End of Study Disposition*

- Global improvement
- Study drug compared with last drug
- Would patient like to continue on study drug
- Reason for early termination
- Disposition for patient management

outcome (Guy 1976), should be used as primary outcome criteria. In patients suffering from panic disorder with or without agoraphobia, scales assessing number and intensity of major panic attacks and phobic avoidance should be used (Ballenger et al. 1988). In antidepressant trials, the rating scales of first choice are the Hamilton Depression Scale (Hamilton 1960), again the CGI global ratings of psychopathology and improvement (Guy 1976), and possibly the Montgomery-Asberg rating scale (Montgomery and Asberg 1979).

It has been found helpful to analyze the ECDEU factors of the Hamilton Depression Scale-21 items (Guy 1976) separately, as well as several "core depression" clusters such as those by Rickels et al. (1987) or Bech et al. (1975). The core depression factor of Rickels et al. includes the following Hamilton Depression items: depressed mood, guilt, suicide, work-activity, retardation, agitation, weight loss, diurnal variation. Also, Rhoades and Overall (1983) reported on a "vegetative depression" and a "cognitive depression" factor of the Hamilton Depression Scale. Finally, D.S. Robinson (personal communication) added three items to the Hamilton Depression Scale, namely hypersomnia, increased appetite, and weight gain.

The Hopkins Symptom Checklist (Derogatis et al. 1974) and the Profile of Mood Scales (POMS) (McNair et al. 1971) are the most frequently used patient-completed rating scales, but other scales are also used, such as the Zung Anxiety (Zung 1971) and Zung Depression (Zung 1965) scales, the Clyde Mood Scale (Clyde 1983), the Beck depression inventory (Beck and Beck 1972), the TSD Scale (Obermaier et al. 1983), and the von Zerssen Beschwerdeliste (von Zerssen 1971). A collection of scales for German-speaking investigators has also been published (CIPS 1981).

It should be remembered that rating scales such as the Hamilton Anxiety and Depression Scales are excellent instruments for measuring change, but they were never designed to make a psychiatric diagnosis. In fact, it is quite possible for a purely anxious GAD patient with no secondary depression to have a Hamilton Depression Scale score $> 18$, simply by endorsing all anxiety and 2 of the 3 sleep items.

In general, most researchers believe that most emphasis should be placed on observer rating and less on patient rating, and that this is particularly true when studying treatments for depression. Our group found it also clinically important to obtain several general global estimates of drug efficacy which, in addition to the usual assessment of global change, should include such questions as "would the patient like to stay on his medication," and for those patients who had drugs prescribed previously, "how was the study drug compared to the last drug the patient had received."

*Side effect assessments* can be conducted either indirectly or specifically, as for example with the Treatment Emergent Symptom Scale (TESS) (Guy 1976) or the SAFTEE (Levine and Schooler 1984). Side effects are identified in terms of severity, duration, whether they necessitated an action by the physician, and whether they are drug-related or not. While some researchers find it useful to read to the patients all items of a given side effect scale at every visit, others do so only at study onset, while still others believe that the concept of "treatment-emergent symptoms" does not necessarily give a true estimate of side effects.

In most studies, side effects are inquired into by an indirect way, with such global questions as "How else did the medication make you feel?" or "Did the medication produce anything negative?" Answers are then recorded either on a checklist or are entered into an adverse event form provided for such assessment. It is recommended that the same adverse event page be used during the whole study, and not a new form each week, necessitating constant referring back and forth between visits. Adverse events are recorded as to intensity, duration, degree of drug relationship, and whether or not they necessitated an intervention.

Downing and Rickels (Downing et al. 1970; Rickels and Downing 1970) examined both side effect assessment methods and concluded that major side effects can be assessed equally well by either method, while mild side effects would be more easily picked up by reading to the patient each possible side effect. The latter approach, however, also led to the assessment of a number of "side effects" such as dandruff, which certainly were not drug-related.

More recently, researchers began to realize that other "adverse events" than side effects need be recorded; for example, if a patient comes down with the flu. Most likely, investigators felt that this would indeed be a medical illness and thus not record it as a side effect. However, more recently, particularly with the experience gained with drugs such as zimelidine and nomifensine, it has become apparent that flu-like symptoms and elevated temperature may well represent drug reactions. Thus, one should not automatically believe that cold or flu-like symptoms represent a medical illness, as conceivably these symptoms may be drug-related.

This example again points to the importance of the inclusion of a placebo group in the research design. If indeed a flu epidemic occurs, flu-like symptoms should appear with equal frequency in both drug and placebo groups; on the other hand, if symptoms are drug-related, they should occur only in the drug group.

It should be mentioned here that more recently, researchers began to realize that *postmarketing surveillance* of new drugs (Mellinger et al. 1988) has an important place in the development of any new medication. This is particularly true for the detection of rare side effects or unsuspected drug interactions, and for the assessment of side effects in the elderly population, which most likely would not have been extensively studied prior to drug approval for marketing.

In drug trials conducted with GAD and PD patients, one should also look for "*rebound anxiety*" by adding a 1-week placebo or no treatment period to the usual 4- to 6-week double-blind acute treatment period (Rickels et al. 1988a). More typical withdrawal reactions lasting longer than a few days are probably not to be expected after such a short period of treatment time, but may occur only after treatment lasting 4–6 months (Rickels et al. 1983, 1988b; Owen and Tyrer 1983). *Withdrawal responses* depend on the daily drug dose taken and the duration of treatment. In studies of 3 to 6 weeks' duration, physical dependence is usually not expected; but rebound anxiety may occur in about 25% of patients treated with short half-life benzodiazepines (Rickels et al. 1988a). Clearly, in studies of 6 months' duration, we have been able to demonstrate significant evidence for the development of physical dependence and the occurrence of clearly measurable withdrawal symptoms in about 40% of patients, even when treated with long half-life benzodiazepines (Rickels et al. 1983, 1988b), but not when treated with the nonbenzodiazepine anxiolytic buspirone (Rickels et al. 1988b).

In antidepressant trials, one may more likely observe an early recurrence of the depression, but withdrawal responses have certainly been reported (Kramer et al. 1961).

### 4.1 Other Safety Assessments

A careful history has to be obtained regarding all concurrent illnesses that may be present during the trial, and all concurrent nonstudy medications being used by the patients, including such over-the-counter medications as cold remedies or aspirin. Compliance with drug taking is assessed by patient inquiry, pill count, and a review of the patient's diary. Reasons for drug intake deviation, as well as for actual medication taken, need to be recorded. Finally, for patients who drop out of the trial, reasons for dropping out should be inquired into and recorded.

Laboratory tests measuring hematology, blood chemistry, urinalysis, and electrocardiograms are conducted at appropriate intervals, both for excluding patients with abnormal values from the drug trial and as an assessment of drug safety during the trial. A full medical examination also needs to be conducted at least pre- and poststudy. Any patients who develop abnormal laboratory or medical signs or values during the study need to be followed poststudy until values have returned to normal or to prestudy levels.

Several years ago, our group introduced the use of a *daily diary* as a measure to improve compliance (Table 7). On this diary, we record for every day how a patient should take his medication, and the patient is asked to record each day how he actually took his study medication, and if he deviated, for what reason. He is also asked to record any possible adverse events, the taking of any concurrent medications and if he did so, for what reasons. For panic patients, a column is added on which the patient records the number and intensity of major panic attacks that he experienced during the past week. Such a diary is used by the physician and rater to review with the patient all information recorded on the form as a help in obtaining the necessary information needed to be transcribed on the weekly study record.

## 5 Study Design

Table 8 lists various design parameters and other methodological issues. Clinical trials should be conducted under double-blind conditions, and patients be assigned to the trial in successive order according to a systematized randomization procedure, which assures equal number of patients for each treatment group to be assigned in relatively small subgroups of patients.

Any design should consider a 1- to 2-week placebo or no-treatment *"run-in" or "washout" period.* If the placebo washout period lasts for only 1 week, an additional 1-week drug-free period should be included for those patients who

**Table 7.** University of Pennsylvania Department of Psychiatry Private Practice Research Group/ Psychopharmacology Research Unit

*Patient Diary*

*Next Appointment:* ____________________

Patient initials: ____________________ Study name: ____________________
Patient number: ____________________ Study week: ____________________

*Introduction:* Please complete daily and bring with you at your next visit. It is not necessary to list those medications taken regularly during the whole study (e.g., birth control pills, medication for hypertension). It is important to return all unused study medication, including empty bottles. Thank you for your cooperation.

| Study Day | Day of Week & Date[a] | Medication prescribed[a] | | Medication Taken | Medication Reason for change | Side effects | Nonstudy medication not mentioned at intake | No. of distinct panic attacks |
|---|---|---|---|---|---|---|---|---|
| | | A.M.: | ______ | ______ | | | | |
| | | NOON: | ______ | ______ | | | | |
| | | P.M.: | ______ | ______ | | | | |
| 1. | | BED: | ______ | ______ | | | | |
| | | A.M.: | ______ | ______ | | | | |
| | | NOON: | ______ | ______ | | | | |
| | | P.M.: | ______ | ______ | | | | |
| 2. | | BED: | ______ | ______ | | | | |
| | | A.M.: | ______ | ______ | | | | |
| | | NOON: | ______ | ______ | | | | |
| | | P.M.: | ______ | ______ | | | | |
| 3. | | BED: | ______ | ______ | | | | |
| | | A.M.: | ______ | ______ | | | | |
| | | NOON: | ______ | ______ | | | | |
| | | P.M.: | ______ | ______ | | | | |
| 4. | | BED: | ______ | ______ | | | | |
| | | A.M.: | ______ | ______ | | | | |
| | | NOON: | ______ | ______ | | | | |
| | | P.M.: | ______ | ______ | | | | |
| 5. | | BED: | ______ | ______ | | | | |
| | | A.M.: | ______ | ______ | | | | |
| | | NOON: | ______ | ______ | | | | |
| | | P.M.: | ______ | ______ | | | | |
| 6. | | BED: | ______ | ______ | | | | |
| | | A.M.: | ______ | ______ | | | | |
| | | NOON: | ______ | ______ | | | | |
| | | P.M.: | ______ | ______ | | | | |
| 7. | | BED: | ______ | ______ | | | | |
| | | A.M.: | ______ | ______ | | | | |
| | | NOON: | ______ | ______ | | | | |
| | | P.M.: | ______ | ______ | | | | |
| 8. | | BED: | ______ | ______ | | | | |
| | | A.M.: | ______ | ______ | | | | |
| | | NOON: | ______ | ______ | | | | |
| | | P.M.: | ______ | ______ | | | | |
| 9. | | BED: | ______ | ______ | | | | |

Total number of capsules (1) dispensed ________ (2) returned ________

[a] Completed before patient leaves office.

Rickels, 3/89.

**Table 8.** Study design

| | |
|---|---|
| *Emphasis on:* | |
| Efficacy | |
| Adverse Events | |
| Tolerance | |
| Relapse | |
| Withdrawal | |
| *Preferred design* | |
| Parallel group design: | Experimental drug |
| | Reference drug |
| | Placebo |
| Placebo a necessity for appropriate efficacy and adverse event assessment | |
| Double-blind, drugs randomized | |
| Several fixed dose comparisons with placebo | |
| Placebo or drug-free run-in (washout) period | |
| *Dosage schedule:* | |
| Fixed dosage | |
| Flexible dosage | |
| Frequency of daily dosing | |
| *Duration:* | |
| Acute: | 2–8 weeks |
| Chronic: | 8–52 weeks |
| *Study sample* | |
| Single/multicenter | |
| Adequate sample size (40–60 per study group) | |
| *Patient protection:* | |
| Parachute clause for worsening, medical illness, suicidal ideation, severe adverse events | |

have been on long half-life psychotropic medications up to the time of study enrollment. Results presented in Table 9 are a good example that a 1-week placebo washout period was not enough to have the long half-life benzodiazepine diazepam eliminated from the plasma. After 1 week of placebo, patients still had significant and measurable levels of diazepam and desmethyldiazepam in their plasma. In contrast, short half-life benzodiazepines such as alprazolam and lorazepam will have been completely eliminated from the plasma in most patients (Rickels et al. in press). For anxiety studies, this washout period is particularly important if one studies "non-benzodiazepine anxiolytics" not cross-tolerant with benzodiazepines. Thus, one has to make sure that benzodiazepine-treated patients do not experience withdrawal symptoms when entering an anxiolytic trial.

A "run-in" or "washout" period is less important for washing out a few placebo responders than for eliminating psychoactive drugs from the system and for allowing the patient to discuss study participation with his or her spouse, to

**Table 9.** Drug plasma levels after a 1-week placebo washout period for patients who took diazepam or clorazepate up to the beginning of the washout period

| | |
|---|---|
| 31 Patients: D+DD plasma level < 400 ng/ml | = 98 ng/ml |
| 11 Patients: D+DD plasma level > 400 ng/ml | = 773 ng/ml |
| 48 Patients: D+DD plasma level | = 281 ng/ml |

think about the frequent "needle sticks" necessary for laboratory tests, and to reflect on the long and frequent travel to the study site, before deciding whether he or she will be committed and motivated enough to participate in the trial and be compliant with the protocol. For study-unrelated reasons, I do encourage dropouts at this time rather than after having entered the patient into the double-blind part of the protocol.

During this "washout" or "run-in" period, the study protocol should allow, however, for occasional use of psychotropic or hypnotic medications, as long as such use is clearly defined in the protocol and recorded by the physician on the appropriate research form.

It certainly goes without saying that one should not initiate large-scale double-blind trials until one is fairly sure about the *effective dosage range* for the experimental drug. Therefore, even in early phase 2 drug development, small open dosage range studies, conducted by a few expert investigators, are important to define the daily dosage range in terms of side effects and improvement. It must be recognized, however, that only placebo-controlled studies will eventually demonstrate whether such improvement observed in an open trial represents a pharmacological or only a placebo response. To be sure about the effective dosage range of an experimental drug is particularly important when one plans to compare the experimental drug, not only against a placebo but against a reference compound. To this end, an investigational program for a new drug should include at least one larger study, comparing several "fixed dosage groups" with each other and with placebo. This method allows us to determine the optimal daily dose that produces the greatest improvement and the least amount of adverse effects in the majority of patients.

Parallel to such fixed dose studies, we suggest that a study with a flexible dosage regimen should also be conducted. One starts with a minimal daily dose and builds this dose up via an obligatory dosage increase regimen rather swiftly until either disturbing side effects occur, the allowable maximum daily dosage is reached, or significant improvement has occurred. The negative aspect of such a trial design is that one may prescribe more medication than the patient actually needs, and thus cause more side effects than are necessary. On the other hand, such design prevents the possible mistake of determining drug inefficacy simply because the daily dosage was too low. Clearly, some guidance about dosage increase must be given to the physician, as physicians tend not to increase medication rigorously unless clearly specified in the design. A good example of a drug development that probably used too-high daily dosages was the one conducted with fluoxetine. Most studies were conducted in the dosage range of 40 to 80 mg/day. Only at the end of fluoxetine's drug development did it become obvious that 20 mg/day of fluoxetine was all the daily medication needed for most depressed patients, also causing fewer side effects than occurred on an 80 mg/day dose.

*Frequency of prescription* during the day depends to a large extent on the half-life of the drug, but also on such factors as how fast the drug is absorbed, how much is protein-bound, how lipophilic the drug is, etc. The less frequently a patient has to take his medication, the better is usually his compliance.

All but possibly the first dosage range study should include a *placebo group*. Our preferred design is a two-way (experimental drug and placebo) or a three-way (experimental drug, reference drug, and placebo) design. For depressed patients, a modified parallel group design is sometimes used. Every patient is treated for 6–8 weeks with the experimental drug and then, under double-blind conditions, either continued on the drug or switched to placebo. Relapse becomes now the main outcome measure. Crossover designs should hardly ever be used in clinical trials of anxiety and depression, as these conditions frequently wax and wane.

As soon as a dosage range for a new drug is fairly well established, three-way studies should be initiated, in which the drug is compared both *against a placebo and a reference drug;* the response to the reference drug and to the placebo serves as a yardstick against which one measures the new drug's response. This is done also to protect the new experimental drug, because if no experimental drug-placebo differences are found, and also none exist between placebo and reference drug, then one is permitted to conclude that the study is inconclusive, representing a waste of resources, but it cannot be counted as a negative study.

But even without a reference drug, if the observed placebo improvement rate is in the 50%–60% rate, a lack of a drug-placebo difference does not necessarily speak against the effectiveness of the experimental drug; rather, such results are again uninterpretable. On the other hand, if both, experimental drug and placebo, produce a response in the 20%–40% range, one would draw the conclusion that one probably has an ineffective compound.

The use of a placebo group may well affect patient selection and the number of weeks a physician is willing to keep an unimproved patient in the study protocol. A physician may assign less ill patients into a placebo trial than he would into a trial which does not include a placebo group. Furthermore, as sponsors interpret the FDA's "70% rule," which states that a study should be analyzed for the duration when at least 70% of the total study populations are still in treatment, as gospel, physicians are frequently forced to keep unimproved placebo and drug patients, or persons experiencing disturbing adverse effects for a prolonged period of time in a trial, long past the time when it would be prudent from a medical and ethical point of view to discontinue such patients. This is an issue of ethical concern with which Institutional Review Boards need to wrestle. This author sees a confrontation between the sponsor and the FDA's desire to have as few dropouts as possible, and the ethical physician and his Institutional Review Board, who need to protect their patients from any possible harm.

I personally do not believe that the FDA is as rigid in regard to the 70% rule as the pharmaceutical industry believes. The FDA itself has recommended the use of parachute clauses in any study utilizing a placebo (Temple 1984). What the FDA quite rightfully views as a design flaw is if patients on a well-accepted reference drug drop out of therapy very early. Such excessive dropout rates on an accepted standard drug would indicate to me, as it probably does to the FDA, that the trial was not conducted in an appropriate and proper manner, and probably also may have used an inappropriate patient population.

With appropriate safety valves or "parachutes," a placebo group is a *must* in clinical drug trials. Many patients do, in fact, improve while on placebo; also, placebo is certainly not toxic, a statement that cannot always be made for an unknown experimental compound (Rickels 1986).

*Length of treatment* is also an important methodologic issue. Studies with anxiolytics should not be carried out for prolonged periods of time, while studies with antidepressants should be carried out for longer periods of time, at least for improved patients.

Some 4–8 weeks is all that is needed to assess drug efficacy in GAD and PD. In fact, most beneficial effects produced by benzodiazepine compounds occur within the first week of treatment (Ballenger et al. 1988; Downing and Rickels 1985). But even for the newer nonbenzodiazepine compounds such as buspirone, efficacy certainly is present after 2–4 weeks of therapy (Rickels et al. 1982, 1988b). Chronic treatment studies should be conducted, similar to those carried out in depression, with chronically anxious patients and patients suffering from PD with or without agoraphobia or other phobic avoidance behavior. Such long-term studies of 4–6 months' duration are needed to address safety and efficacy questions (Rickels et al. 1988b). Some of these long-term studies may simply be added on to acute studies, using either a single- or double-blind methodology, while others are specially designed, including a double-blind switch to placebo after chronic treatment, to assess incidence and severity of rebound anxiety and/or physical dependence (Rickels et al. 1983, 1988b). The author strongly urges not to carry out studies in anxiety for periods longer than 6 months, as the vast majority of anxious patients would be unnecessarily exposed to prolonged drug use. While many chronic patients may need anxiolytics intermittently for years, hardly any patient needs anxiolytics continuously (Rickels 1983; Rickels et al. 1986).

In depression, longer treatment periods are frequently appropriate. Most clinicians feel that probably 3–6 months of maintenance therapy is appropriate, even for patients with a first single episode of major depression. Thus, as soon as possible, it would be important to build into any acute trial with antidepressants lasting 6–8 weeks the option, still under double-blind conditions, to maintain improved patients in a chronic maintenance phase for 6–12 months.

The problem with most long-term maintenance studies, besides a significant incidence of attrition, is that one never is sure about the percent of patients who are still in need of such therapy and who are not. Figure 1 provides a possible design to answer this haunting question (Rickels et al. 1983). One-third of patients are treated with active medication for 6 weeks (acute), one-third for 16 weeks

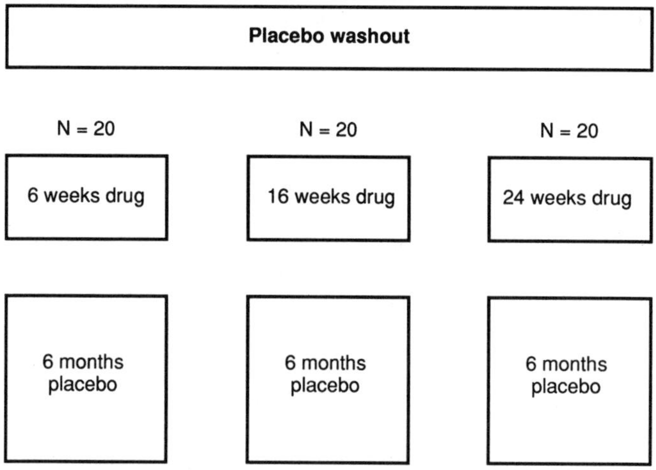


**Fig. 1.** Long-term treatment design. Dropouts followed after 3 and 6 months for (a) emotional state, (b) any therapeutic intervention. After 6 weeks of single-blind drug therapy, the double-blind part starts with 20 patients being shifted to placebo and 40 continuing on drug

(sub-chronic), and one-third for 24 weeks (chronic). Each active drug treatment group is shifted for 6 months, under double-blind conditions, to placebo.

This design should allow for the assessment of: (a) rebound anxiety, which may occur after placebo substitution in the 6-week treated group; (b) typical withdrawal symptoms (Rickels et al. 1983, 1988b; Owen and Tyrer 1983) lasting a few weeks in patients treated for 4 and 6 months with active drug; and (c) return of anxiety or depression. If, for example, every patient who was treated for 6 months remained well for several months while on placebo, such patient probably would not have needed 6 months of drug therapy.

The research questions addressed in chronic therapy usually are:

1. Does prolonged therapy further improve efficacy above that experienced during 6 weeks of acute therapy?
2. Is efficacy maintained without the development of tolerance?
3. Is safety maintained?
4. Do withdrawal symptoms occur upon discontinuation?

*Pharmacokinetics* provide a great deal of information about the drug's half-life and therefore about how the drug should be used. But while drug plasma concentrations correlate highly with daily dose, they usually do not correspond closely with clinical improvement (Rickels et al. 1984). However, if drug plasma concentrations can be easily assessed, they may be employed in those patients who are poor responders despite receiving high daily dosages and without experiencing side effects, and in those patients reporting side effects while on extremely low drug dosages.

Anxiolytic agents, in this author's opinion at least, should also be studied in situational reactions or adjustment reactions prescribed for only a few days.

Emergency rooms may provide appropriate sites. Patients could be followed 2 or 3 days later. Such short-term studies would provide important information not presently available.

One comment may be in order here about the timeframe in which studies need to be conducted. Sponsors frequently demand short timeframes and correspondingly exert excessive pressures on investigators to enroll patients. Those investigators who give in to the sponsor's pressure often, knowingly or not, relax their study intake criteria and enroll patients into a study whom they otherwise would have rejected. Our group accepts as study patients only about one fourth of those screened for possible trial participation. To lower intake standards certainly would yield more patients, but possibly at the cost of loss of sensitivity in detecting drug-placebo differences, by relaxing diagnostic criteria, enrolling patients suffering from Axis II personality disorders, or enrolling noncompliant patients.

Finally, a drug evaluation program should include a battery of *psychomotor tests,* the experimental drug given at several dosage levels, and being compared with a standard drug and with placebo. Usually, such studies can initially be carried out with healthy volunteers, but eventually should include anxious or depressed patients receiving medications under acute and chronic administration (Johnson and Chernik 1982). It is important to study these psychomotor, cognitive and memory effects in dosages normally prescribed to patients and not only in excessively high dosages.

## 6 Statistical Planning and Data Handling

Table 10 touches on some of the design factors to be considered in planning a critical drug evaluation program. The statistician should be involved from the beginning. Before planning a drug trial, one *should predict expected results,* set up a hypothesis, and make specific stipulations of what results will be considered as an acceptable and meaningful measure of outcome. This is particularly true when a variety of rating scales are being used, as some significant findings could simply be expected by chance alone. For example, in anxiety trials, a 50% change in the Hamilton Anxiety Scale total score, a change of at least 2 points on the 7-point CGI Psychopathology Scale, and a moderate and marked but not minimal global improvement could represent such outcome criteria.

For depression trials, one simply replaces the Hamilton Anxiety with the Hamilton Depression scale, and possibly adds the Montgomery-Asberg scale. For panic disorder trials, one chooses the decrease in number and intensity of panic attacks and decrease in phobic avoidance behavior as pivotal outcome measures.

Completer, decreasing sample size as well as endpoint analyses should be conducted for all time periods, applying, whenever appropriate, parametric statistics (Levine et al. 1971; Levine 1979; Overall 1987). The first set of analyses includes only patients who completed the total study period. The second set of analyses uses all patients evaluated at each visit, i.e., a sample size with a

**Table 10.** Statistical planning and data handling

*A*

- Drug randomization
- Double blinding
- Adequate sample size to provide sufficient power to test hypothesis
- Determination of alpha level to be accepted as significant
- Specify size of treatment to be considered clinically significant
- Specify prior to study onset the major outcome criteria and minimum treatment period to be acceptable

*B*

- Parametric and nonparametric tests
- Univariate and multivariate procedures
- Factorial Anovas or Anacovas
- Predictor analyses (multiple regression, discriminant functions, logistic regression)
- Appropriate handling of attrition
- Use of completer, decreasing *n*, and last location carried forward (LOCF; endpoint) analyses

*C*

- Pooling of data across studies
- Single vs multicenter trials

*D*

- Data reporting

decreasing *n*. The third set of analyses is a "last location carried forward" (LOCF), or endpoint analysis, which for anxiety drugs, should include all patients with at least 1-week double-blind treatment, and for depression studies, only patients with at least 2 weeks double-blind treatment. Again, these criteria should be decided before the study is conducted and should be recorded in the protocol. Finally, the FDA requests an "intent to treat analysis," which includes all patients who have received double-blinded medication and for whom one posttreatment assessment is available. The more consistency there is in patterns of response between these various analyses, the more robust are the study results.

When planning a clinical trial, choosing a large enough *sample size* to demonstrate treatment differences is of utmost importance. In calculating study sample size, the investigator must decide what minimal clinical difference in outcome between the experimental and control group he considers clinically significant. The required sample size is usually derived by combining four essential elements, namely type 1 error, type 2 error, minimally accepted magnitude of difference, and estimate of outcome variance of the control group (Dixon and Massey 1969; Feinstein 1977).

Generally speaking, 30–40 patients per group represent the minimum sample size needed to demonstrate significant outcome differences between established antianxiety or antidepressant agents and placebo, and most researchers demand sample sizes of 60 each, while much larger samples are needed when comparing two active agents. In order to obtain large sample sizes of 100–150 patients per group for drug-drug comparisons, one has to combine data from several studies. It is therefore important that these studies use an identical protocol. Also, before initiating a group of multicenter studies (studies that use identical protocols), it has to be clearly stated whether or not these studies are designed as single studies never to be combined, as single studies later to be combined with two or three other single studies, or are only designed as multicenter studies never intended to stand on their own. In general, single-center, large-scale studies are preferred to a multicenter trial. In a multicenter trial, several large individual sites are usually preferred to many small individual sites. This is particularly true if one wants to analyze separately each individual site, if one wants to test for individual site x treatment interactions, or if one wants to statistically block out site effects.

Many small individual sites are preferred in multicenter trials if one wants to generate a study most likely to represent a field trial. However, such a study is only possible if all investigators and raters have worked closely together for many years, and if such a study is clearly supervised by a central group such as our Private Practice Research Group (Rickels et al. 1977). Studies in which drugs are simply distributed to many unrelated different sites, with various degrees of inexperience in research, are certainly not preferable to fewer but larger multicenter sites.

Multicenter trials are thus frequently necessary to provide the sample requirements for a study within an acceptable timeframe; such multicenter trials, however, should not consist of too large a sample size because in this case even a small, clinically insignificant difference between placebo and drug might become statistically significant. Thus, excessive sample sizes in multicenter trials may constitute a waste of valuable resources in terms of funds, time, patients and research staff.

The matter of combining data across several studies is a complex one (Levine 1979; Overall 1987; Overall and Rhoades 1987) and cannot be discussed here in detail. One may combine statistical data such as chi squares or Student's *t*-tests, for example, or one may combine raw data. Such data combining depends to a large extent on whether significant drug/setting interactions in outcome are found. It certainly does not make much clinical sense to combine data from studies which have produced diametrically opposed results (significant setting/treatment interactions). The combining of data is particularly important if one wants to search for possible predictors of improvement, or for subgroups of patients who may respond particularly well or particularly poorly to a given drug treatment.

One comment regarding "pivotal versus nonpivotal" studies. "Pivotal" studies are those studies which the sponsor submits to the FDA or to other drug-approving agencies as providing significant proof that the drug is clinically effective and safe. "Nonpivotal" studies include those which show changes in the same direction as pivotal studies, but these changes may be of no statistical or only trend significance and most studies that do not include a placebo. These latter studies are mainly of interest for the comparison of side effects between drugs and for marketing purposes.

This author also believes that clinical research trial methodology would not suffer if freed from some of the "bureaucratic irritants" usually suggested by the sponsor's data-handling department and not necessarily by the FDA or other drug-regulation agencies.

For example, in a U.S. research study, a physician today spends about 80% of his time on "data recording," including, for example, the day of the week in a given month in a given year that a patient had experienced the onset of a prior psychiatric episode 10 years ago, and in keeping independent visit records separate from study records. Only 20% of the physician's time is spent in what this author considers to be the most important aspect of clinical research, namely the assessment of efficacy and safety. In addition, much of the data recorded in U.S. trials are never fully utilized by the sponsor, never reported in publications, and frequently not even used by the industry in their NDA submission.

Also, minor study violations such as the occasional, random use of psychotropic medications during the study or during the placebo washout period, should not necessarily invalidate the results of a drug trial. An effective experimental drug will always prove to be effective; and an ineffective drug will stay ineffective. In fact, whenever we have analyzed studies including and excluding such minor study violators, we have never observed any significant effect of such violations on study outcome. And, in fact, this is what the FDA obtains from the sponsor when requesting "intent to treat" data analyses.

Finally, *research results have to be reported* in a clear and scientific manner so that the reader not only is able to understand what went on in the study, but will be able to attempt a replication of the study results if he so desires. The report of study results of any drug trial should include the purpose and specific aims of the study, a description and justification of the methods used, and an ample description of the patient sample and of all outcome assessment methods used. Efficacy and adverse event results should be displayed over time and not only for one posttreatment period.

## 7 Conclusion

This chapter discussed several elements relevant for the planning, execution, analysis, and reporting of results of clinical trials conducted with anxiolytics and antidepressants. Certainly there are many other aspects of clinical trial methodology important for the evaluation of psychotropic agents in addition to those discussed here. Nevertheless, it is hoped that this chapter offers some guidance to those interested in the evaluation of anxiolytic and antidepressant agents.

## References

Aitken RCB (1969) Measurement of feeling using visual analogue scales. Proc R Soc Med 62:989–993
American Psychiatric Association (1987) Diagnostic and statistical manual of mental disorders: DSM-III-R. American Psychiatric Association, Washington DC
Ballenger JC, Burrows GD, DuPont RL, Lessner IM, Noyes R, Pecknold JC, Rifkin A, Swinson RP (1988) Alprazolam in panic disorder and agoraphobia: results from a multicenter trial. I. Efficacy in short-term treatment. Arch Gen Psychiatry 45:413–422
Bech P, Gram LF, Dein E, Jacobsen O, Vitger J, Balwig TG (1975) Quantitative rating of depressive states. Acta Psychiatr Scand 51:161–170
Beck AT, Beck RW (1972) Screening depressed patients in family practice. Postgrad Med 52:81
CIPS (1981) Internationale Scalen für Psychiatrie. Beltz-Test, Weinheim
Clyde DJ (1983) Clyde mood scale manual. Clyde Computing Services, Key Largo
Derogatis LR, Lipman RS, Rickels K, Uhlenhuth EH, Covi L (1974) The Hopkins symptom checklist (HSCL): a self-report system inventory. Behav Sci 19:1–15
Dixon WJ, Massey FJ (1969) Introduction of statistical analysis, 3rd edn. McGraw-Hill New York
Downing RW, Rickels K (1981) Coffee consumption, cigarette smoking and the reporting of drowsiness in anxious patients treated with benzodiazepines or placebo. Acta Psychiatr Scand 64:398–408
Downing RW, Rickels K (1985) Early treatment response in anxious outpatients treated with diazepam. Acta Psychiatr Scand 72:522–528
Downing RW, Rickels K, Meyers F (1970) Side reactions in neurotics: I. A comparison of two methods of assessment. J Clin Pharmacol 10:289–297
Endicott J, Spitzer RL (1978) A diagnostic interview: the schedule for affective disorders and schizophrenia. Arch Gen Psychiatry 35:837–844
FDA (1977) General considerations for the clinical evaluation of drugs. Government Printing Office, Washington DC (publ no 77-3040
FDA (1978) Guidelines for the clinical evaluation of psychotropic drugs – antidepressant and antianxiety drugs. Psychopharmacol Bull 14:45–63
Feinstein AR (1977) Clinical biostatistics. Mosby, St Louis, pp 320–334
Goldberg SC (1987) Persistent flaws in the design and analysis of psychopharmacology research. In: Meltzer HY (ed) Psychopharmacology: the third generation of progress. Raven, New York, pp 1005–1012
Guy W (1976) Early clinical drug evaluation program (ECDEV). Assessment manual of psychopharmacology. Department of Health, Education and Welfare, Rockville
Hamilton M (1959) The assessment of anxiety states by rating. Br J Med Psychol 32:50–55
Hamilton M (1960) A rating scale for depression. J Neurol Neurosurg Psychiatry 23:56–62
Johnson LC, Chernik DA (1982) Sedative-hypnotics and human performance. Psychopharmacology 76:101–113
Kramer JC, Klein DF, Fink M (1961) Withdrawal symptoms following discontinuation of imipramine therapy. Am J Psychiatry 118:549–550
Levine J (ed) (1979) Coordinating clinical trials in psychopharmacology. Planning, documentation and analysis. US Government Printing Office, Washington DC pp 63–86
Levine J, Ban TA (1987) Assessment methods in clinical trials. In: Metlzer HY (ed) Psychopharmacology: the third generation of progress. Raven New York, pp 997–1003
Levine J, Schooler NR (1984) SAFTEE (Systematic assessment for treatment emergent events) – a new technique for detecting side effects in clinical trials. Clin Neuropharmacol 7:856–857
Levine J, Schiele BC, Bouthilet L (eds) (1971) Principles and problems of establishing the efficacy of psychotropic agents. US Public Health Service, Washington DC, pp 321–369 (publ no 2138)
Lipman R, Covi L (1976) Outpatient treatment of neurotic depression: medication and group psychotherapy. In: Spitzer RL, Klein DL (eds) Evaluation of the psychological therapies. Johns Hopkins University Press, Baltimore
McNair DM, Lorr M, Droppleman LF (1971) Manual of the profile of mood states. Educational and Industrial Testing Service, San Diego
Mellinger GD, Balter MB, Abramowitz S, Schaffer CB, Bernstein L (1988) Survey method of post-marketing drug surveillance: a demonstration. J Clin Psychopharmacol 8:168–176

Montgomery SA, Asberg M (1979) A new depression scale designed to be sensitive to change. Br J Psychiatry 134:382–389
Obermaier W, Rickels K, Stoll KD (1983) Test zur Erfassung der Schwere einer Depression (TSD). Manual Beltz Test, Weinheim
Overall JE (1987) Introduction: methodology in psychopharmacology. In: Meltzer HY (ed) Psychopharmacology: the third generation of progress. Raven, New York, pp 995–996
Overall JE, Rhoades HM (1987) Adjusting *p* values for multiple tests of significance. In: Meltzer HY (ed) Psychopharmacology: the third generation of progress. Raven, New York, pp 1013–1018
Owen RT, Tyrer P (1983) Benzodiazepine dependence – a review of the evidence. Drugs 25:385–398
Raskin A, Schulterbrandt JG, Reatig N, McKeon JJ (1970) Differential response to chlorpromazine, imipramine, and placebo. Arch Gen Psychiatry 23:164–173
Rhoades HM, Overall JE (1983) The Hamilton depression scale: factor scoring and profile classification. Psychopharmacol Bull 19:91–96
Rickels K (ed) (1968) Non-specific factors in drug therapy. Thomas, Springfield
Rickels K (1983) Benzodiazepines in the treatment of anxiety: North American experiences. In: Costa E (ed) The benzodiazepines: from molecular biology to clinical practice. Raven, New York, pp 295–310
Rickels K (1986) Use of placebo in clinical trials. Psychopharmacol Bull 22:93–99
Rickels K, Downing RW (1970) Side reactions in neurotics: II. Can patients judge which symptoms are caused by their medication? J Clin Pharmacol 10:298–305
Rickels K, Hesbacher P, Fisher EL, Norstad N (1977) The private practice research group (PPRG): a working model from psychopharmacology for clinical research in family practice. J Clin Pharmacol 17:541–554
Rickels K, Wiseman K, Norstad N, Singer M, Stoltz D, Brown A, Danton J (1982) Buspirone and diazepam in anxiety: a controlled study. J Clin Psychiatry 43:81–86
Rickels K, Case GW, Downing RW, Winokur A (1983) Long-term diazepam therapy and clinical outcome. JAMA 250:767–771
Rickels K, Case WG, Downing RW, Dixon R, Fridman R (1984) Diazepam and desmethyldiazepam plasma concentrations in chronic anxious outpatients. Pharmacopsychiatry 17:44–49
Rickels K, Case WG, Downing RW, Fridman R (1986) One-year follow-up of anxious patients treated with diazepam. J Clin Psychopharmacol 6:32–36
Rickels K, Chung HR, Csanalosi IB, Hurowitz AM, London J, Wiseman K, Kaplan M, Amsterdam JD (1987) Alprazolam, diazepam, imipramine, and placebo in outpatients with major depression. Arch Gen Psychiatry 44:862–866
Rickels K, Fox IL, Greenblatt DJ, Sandler KR, Schless A (1988a) Chlorazepate and lorazepam: clinical improvement and rebound anxiety. Am J Psychiatry 145:312–317
Rickels K, Schweizer E, Csanalosi I, Case WG, Chung H (1988b) Long-term treatment of anxiety and risk of withdrawal: prospective comparison of clorazepate and buspirone. Arch Gen Psychiatry 45:444–450
Rickels K, Schweizer E, Case WG, Greenblatt D, Chronic therapeutic use of benzodiazepines. I. Effects of abrupt discontinuation. Arch Gen Psychiatry (in press)
Sartorius N, Jablensky A, Cooper JE, Burke JD (eds) (1988) Psychiatric classification in an international perspective. Br J Psychiatry 152 [Suppl 1]:
Spitzer RL, Williams JW (1983) Instruction manual for the structured clinical interview for DSM-III (SCID). Revision Biometrics Research Department, New York State Psychiatric Institute, New York
Spitzer RL, Endicott JD, Robins E (1978) Research diagnostic criteria: rationale and reliability. Arch Gen Psychiatry 35:773–782
Temple R (1984) Current issues in the design, conduct, and interpretation of clinical trials. Workshop Proceedings, Washington DC, 10 September 1984
von Zerssen D (1971) Die Beschwerdeliste als Test. Therapiewoche 21:1908–1914
Wittenborn JR (ed) (1977) Guidelines for clinical trials of psychotropic drugs. Pharmakopsychiatrie Neuro-Psychopharmakol 10:205–231
Zung WWK (1965) A self-rating depression scale. Arch Gen Psychiatry 12:63–70
Zung WWK (1971) A rating instrument for anxiety disorders. Psychosomatics 12:271–279

# Testing the Efficacy of New Neuroleptic Drugs

S.R. HIRSCH and T.R.E. BARNES[1]

A new era in the treatment of psychosis may be heralded by the recent appearance of compounds which are active in the treatment of psychosis yet have radically different pharmacological properties from those antipsychotic drugs currently available. Some of these compounds lack the rapid sedative action which characterises existing neuroleptics, and the clinical psychopharmacologist faces a real problem in evaluating the antipsychotic efficacy of these novel, non-sedative drugs.

## 1 Requirements of Drug Licensing Authorities

A basic requirement of all drug licensing authorities is that a new treatment is shown to be both effective and safe. The principal strategy adopted to demonstrate that a drug is effective is either to show that it is superior to placebo or to show that it is as good as established treatments. In some countries, such as the United States, drug administration authorities are reluctant to license new drugs that cannot be demonstrated to have some advantage over drugs already on the market. In this case one must show either that the drug is more effective therapeutically than existing medication or that it produces fewer or less severe side effects.

This paper discusses the practical problems of placebo-controlled studies, in the knowledge that they remain the most rapid and efficient way to demonstrate that a drug has a specific clinical effect. The numbers required are relatively small – for example in order to show that a treatment with an observed improvement rate of 65%-70% is significantly better than placebo, with an improvement rate of 25%-35%, a minimum of 17 patients need be treated in each group ($P < .05$) (Day and Graham 1989). Further, the difference between the improvement rate on placebo and the experimental treatment gives a direct measure of the specific pharmacological effect of the new treatment over and above nonspecific effects observed under placebo.

[1] Charing Cross and Westminster Medical School, University of London, Department of Psychiatry, Fulham Palace Road, London W6, United Kingdom

**Methodology of the Evaluation of Psychotropic Drugs**
Editors: O. Benkert, W. Maier, and K. Rickels
(Psychopharmacology Series 8)
© Springer-Verlag Berlin Heidelberg 1990

## 2 Is Establishing Efficacy by Comparison with a Standard Drug a Practical Approach?

It is sometimes considered more practicable to establish the efficacy of a new treatment for a particular disorder by comparing it with a treatment which is already known to be effective. In practice this may not be so because of the large number of patients required if a type II error is to be avoided. That is to say, if two treatments appear to be equally effective, a statistical test of "power" must be used to rule out the possibility that the apparent similarity between the two treatments is not a mere matter of chance, that is, to reduce the risk of concluding there is no difference when there really is a difference (Hirsch and Macrae 1986; Day and Graham 1989). In order to exclude the possibility that an observed difference of 20% or less between two treatments is not a matter of chance at the 95% confidence level (power = 0.95), one would need 154 patients in each group, if the improvement rate for one of the two treatments was 70%, and 161 patients in each group if the improvement rate in one of the two treatments was 60%. In order to show that no more than a 10% difference between the two treatments could occur by chance at the 95% confidence level, one would need 589 patients in each group if the response rate on one of the treatments was 70%, and 641 if the response rate was 60%. With patient groups smaller than these there would be little scientific justification for concluding that the lack of significant difference between a new treatment and a standard treatment demonstrated that the new treatment was as good as the standard one.

There are other problems in relying on a comparison between two active treatments. First, the improvement which is observed in each treatment, even if identical, may be simply due to the passage of time and the natural course of the disorder. Thus, a pharmacological effect cannot be demonstrated scientifically by comparing one treatment with another if the two have the same apparent effect. If such a comparison shows one treatment to be significantly different from another then there is a problem of interpretation. For example, the observed difference could be due to a failure to use clinically equivalent doses of the two drugs. Many studies which find that one drug is more efficacious or has fewer side effects than another are due to a failure in matching clinically effective doses. Dosage equivalents of neuroleptics have been determined by a number of methods, including in vitro studies of their potency in blocking H3 spiroperidol binding (Creese et al. 1976; Seeman et al. 1976), differences in their tendency to cause extrapyramidal side effects, and the dosage of the drug which has proved effective in establishing the drug's treatment superiority over placebo as a ratio to the corresponding dosage of chlorpromazine (Davis 1976). However, these three methods do not correlate so well that one can view them as interchangeable and each leads to slightly different determinations of dosage equivalents.

## 3 Constraints on Clinical Trials of New Neuroleptics

If comparing a new drug with a standard treatment is not an efficient way to determine the efficacy of a new drug, are there serious difficulties with placebo-controlled studies? The most common question which clinicians and pharmaceutical companies seek to answer is whether a drug provides an effective treatment in acute illness. In acute episodes, treatment response is easily discernible and every medication which has proved effective in preventing relapse and maintaining patients outside hospital in the long-term has always been effective in treating the acute phase of psychosis. Unfortunately, acute patients not infrequently refuse medication and have to be treated compulsorily. In many countries it would be considered unethical as well as impractical and possibly illegal to treat a legally restrained patient in hospital with a placebo, randomly allocated in the context of a placebo-controlled drug trial. Other patients who are prepared to have the standard treatment may refuse to have an unproven treatment or be part of an experimental trial. Of equal or greater importance is the reluctance on the part of nurses and doctors to allow their patients to participate in a study in which they may receive placebo medication. The clinical team may fear that a patient on placebo may be unmanageable and violent, or the staff may require assurance that the patients entered into the trial will not present unpredictable difficulties or be denied relief of distressing symptoms. These difficulties are then compounded if the new treatment which may be a good antipsychotic is nevertheless not sedative and takes 1 or 2 weeks to bring a patient's illness under control.

## 4 Which Patients Are Available for Acute Treatment Studies of Antipsychotics?

Who then gets excluded from acute treatment trials? Patients who are suicidal, over-active, or agitated; patients who are threatening or violent; patients who are suffering or distressed by their symptoms; patients who are too paranoid to cooperate; and anyone who is likely to be a management problem at a time when the ward has too many other patients who are management problems.

Who then are the patients generally available for acute placebo studies? They are likely to be patients who are mildly ill, very chronic patients with symptoms which have not responded to other treatments, or patients who have found previous treatments unacceptable because of side effects. None of these cases is appropriate for testing the efficacy of a new antipsychotic drug if we are interested in its effect on common and representative types of problems.

In practice, a very few selected patients are found to be suitable for drug treatment studies. For example, in our initial attempts to compare the efficacy of propranolol to placebo in the treatment of acute psychosis (Manchanda and Hirsch 1986), we only managed to recruit two patients in the first 18 months.

However, if one *is* able to overcome the objections we have just identified for placebo-controlled studies, individual patients often see advantages in being in such a trial, even those who are being compulsorily detained for treatment. Participation in the trial guarantees close clinical monitoring by the investigators and careful measurement of the effects of the treatment. There is less risk of precipitant treatment before the diagnosis has been accurately determined. Patients and their families are able to appreciate the advantage of determining if they are among the 20% or so of patients who will improve without drugs and if patients are assigned to placebo, it will be possible to make some assessment of whether or not they really needed active treatment. By being in a placebo-controlled trial they have a chance to avoid being treated with active medication, a fact which is satisfying to those who wish to avoid treatment altogether but know the alternative is to have active medication compulsorily. Given that another 20% or so of patients do not respond to standard treatment, the opportunity of receiving a new treatment which may be more efficacious or have fewer side effects also has an appeal. Finally, both the patients and the clinicians would be reassured to know that research has indicated that there is no long-term disadvantage in being treated with placebo in a drug trial, even if this is associated with a relapse. This was the result of a 7-year follow-up study we carried out of an earlier placebo substitution study which first determined the efficacy of fluphenazine decanoate depot medication in the late 1960s (Curson et al. 1986; Hirsch et al. 1973).

## 5 Modified Acute Placebo-Controlled Design

We have developed a modification of the placebo-controlled design which we have found overcomes most of the objections to the use of placebos in acute clinical studies but retains most of the advantages (Manchanda and Hirsch 1986). We had wanted to establish whether propranolol has any pharmacological effect on the symptoms of acute schizophrenia, using a standard placebo-controlled trial design. However, as stated above we had only recruited two patients in 18 months. We then modified the design so that all patients had haloperidol 10 mg per day for the first week as well as either propranolol or placebo on a randomised basis. After the first week, haloperidol was withdrawn and patients continued on either propranolol or placebo for the next 3 weeks (see Fig. 1). In addition to the end-point analysis whenever the patients withdrew from the trial, the number of patients dropping out in each group and the number of patients receiving additional medication as an adjunct – either valium or short-acting neuroleptics – were used as dependent outcome variables. Significantly more patients dropped out from the placebo-treated group and there was a significantly greater deterioration in symptoms from the end of the first week to the end of the fourth week in patients treated with placebo, compared with those receiving propranolol.

Haloperidol was resumed from week 4 to week 8, although this is not shown in Fig. 1. The rate of improvement on haloperidol was much greater than with either placebo or propranolol. The study demonstrated that propranolol had a significant pharmacological effect, although from a clinical point of view it was not very useful.

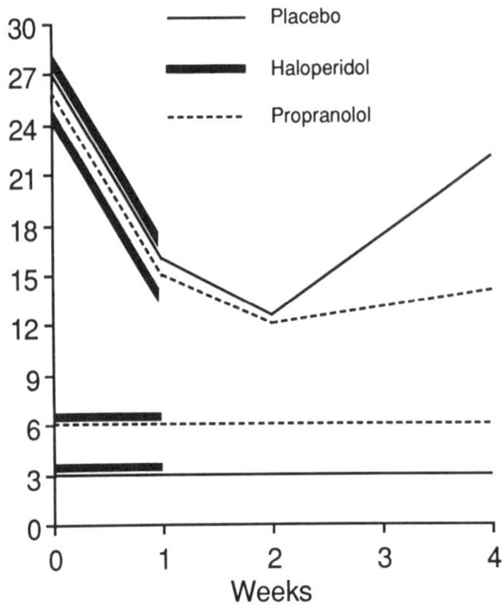


**Fig. 1.** Comparison of placebo, haloperidol, and propranolol in acute schizophrenia: total BPRS score

The validity of this approach is reinforced in Fig. 2 which compares the results on the non-thought disordered schizophrenia sub-scale of the Brief Psychiatric Rating Scale (BPRS) (Overall and Gorham 1962) for patients on placebo and propranolol from weeks 1 to 4. Figure 3 shows the non-schizophrenia sub-scales of the BPRS in the two groups. These figures reveal that non-thought disordered schizophrenic symptoms deteriorated in patients on placebo but not those on propranolol between weeks 1 and 4, but non-specific symptoms not related directly to schizophrenia deteriorated as much in the propranolol-treated group as in the placebo group.

Figure 4 illustrates the modified design we would recommend if the new drug under test has powerful sedative properties. In this case, patients could be randomised on a two-way basis between the experimental treatment (new drug) plus placebo haloperidol from the start of the treatment, and a combination of placebo plus 10 mg of haloperidol or an equivalent neuroleptic for the first week in the control group, followed by placebo only for the next 3 weeks in the control group. Both groups would receive the standard neuroleptic for the second 4 weeks in order to examine whether the slope of improvement is greater on the standard neuroleptic than placebo or the experimental treatment. If a sufficient number of patients are available, one refinement would be a third treatment group who have the standard neuroleptic throughout. This would allow comparison of the new treatment with the standard treatment, and assessment of whether the new and standard treatment are significantly better than placebo, thereby indicating that the patients were essentially responsive to treatment. This is especially important if there is no impressive difference between the experimental and standard treatment.

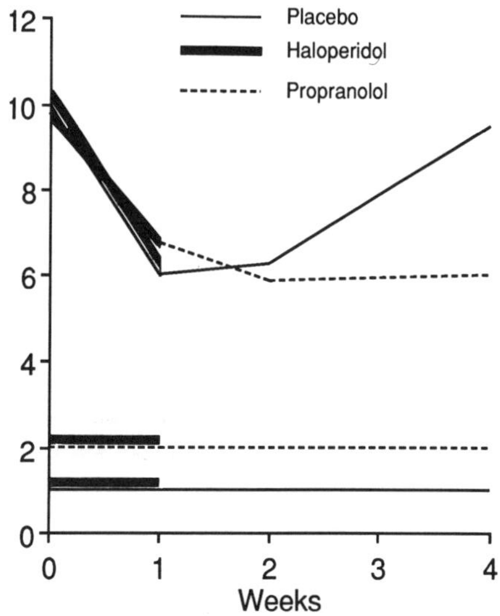


**Fig. 2.** Comparison of placebo, haloperidol, and propranolol in acute schizophrenia: BPRS schizophrenia subscale score

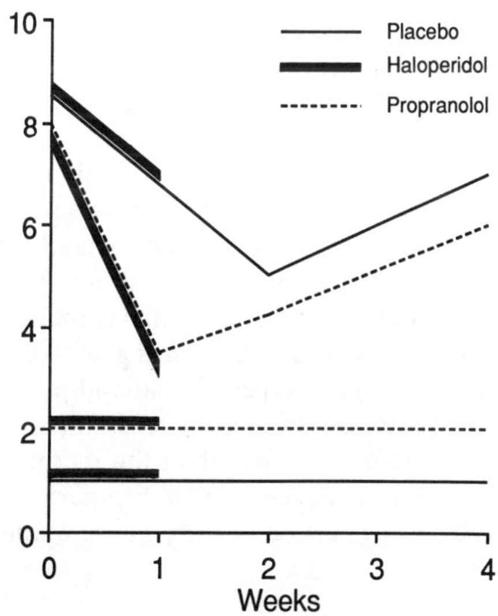


**Fig. 3.** Comparison of placebo, haloperidol, and propranolol in acute schizophrenia: BPRS non-schizophrenia subscale score

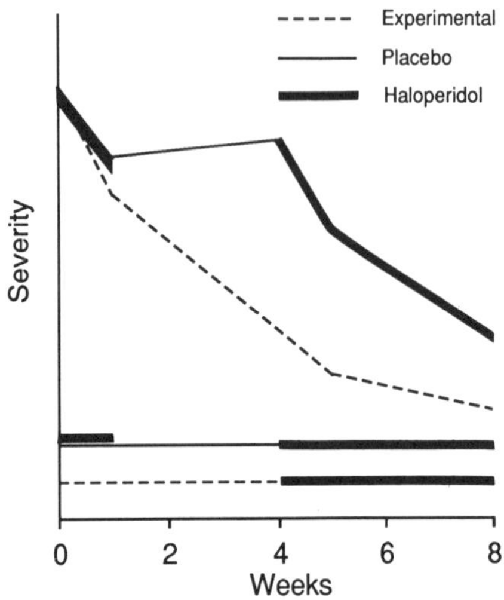


**Fig. 4.** Modified design for a comparative treatment study in acute schizophrenia, testing a sedative experimental drug

## 5.1 Advantages to the Modified Design

The main advantage of the proposed trial design is that all patients receive active treatment, and no patients are treated with placebo alone during the initial week of the study. We found that most patients settle by the end of the first week of haloperidol treatment, but if a disturbance occurs they can either be given adjunct therapy (a benzodiazepine or, if necessary, a short-acting neuroleptic such as droperidol) or they can be withdrawn from the trial. Either intervention provides useful information about the ability of the drug under test to control certain kinds of behaviour.

The more conservative design, and the one that should be used if the experimental drug does not have sedative properties, combines haloperidol plus either placebo or the experimental drug in the first week, followed by placebo or the experimental drug for the following 3 weeks, respectively (Fig. 5). Since a minimum of only 17 patients is required for each treatment group, it might be possible to include a control group receiving standard neuroleptic treatment in addition to the experimental and placebo treatment groups.

In our experience the recruitment rate for this modified design type of study is as great or greater than the recruitment rate for the study on which we are currently engaged, which compares a standard neuroleptic with a new neuroleptic as part of an early phase 2 study.

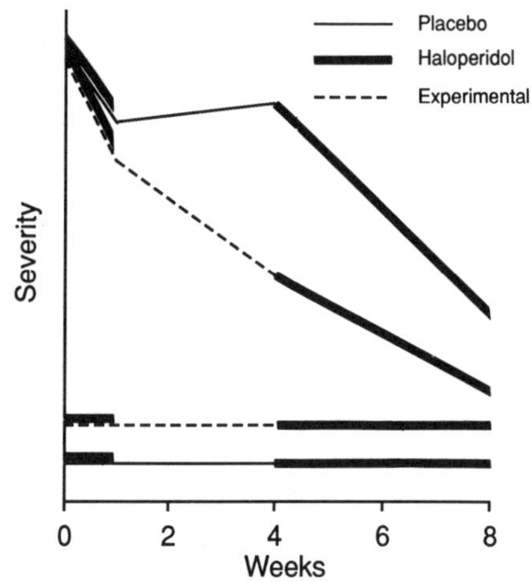


**Fig. 5.** Modified design for a comparative treatment study in acute schizophrenia, testing a non-sedative experimental drug

## 6 Other Approaches for Establishing the Efficacy of New Neuroleptics

Another way of obviating the need for a placebo treatment group is to carry out a study testing for optimum dose level, using a range of doses from very low to very high. Comparing the various dosage groups, one would look for a differential rate of improvement or an indicator of effectiveness. In practice, four groups would probably be necessary for such a study. To be ethically acceptable it should be carried out early in phase II when there is usually uncertainty about the effective dose, although one will be limited at this time by the amount of toxicological data available which will probably not include information on high dosage. The number of patients required for such a study is high as the differences in the magnitude of change between patients receiving medium and low doses are likely to be small as compared with the differences between active drug and placebo.

## 7 Chronic States

The term "chronic schizophrenia" is used to cover patients without persisting disabilities, those with only mild handicaps, who tend to relapse, and patients with moderate or severe refractory symptoms. The symptoms may include only positive symptoms such as delusions, hallucinations and thought disorder (disordered speech), or persistent negative symptoms, including poverty of the content of speech, poverty of the amount of speech, poverty of affect (or flat affect), and poverty of initiative and drive. Many patients in an institutional or unchanging social setting may not express their positive symptoms, although they are usually easily elicited if they are looked for. Even thought disorder may be a symptom which only occurs when the patient is appropriately stimulated.

Because of the variety of medication and medicaments exhibited in any heterogeneous group of chronic patients, it is easier to study the effect of a new drug by using it as an adjunct to standard treatment, in comparison with a placebo adjunct. However, a design in which patients are treated with only the experimental or control treatment gives a more straightforward clinical result. The fact that Kane and others (1988) have recently shown that clozapine is superior to chlorpromazine in the treatment of patients with refractory chronic schizophrenic symptoms, sets a standard for study design and methodology which any trials of new drugs will have to try to emulate.

The distinction between positive and negative symptoms does not provide any new problems for the study of chronic patients other than the need to choose a scale which adequately measures the range of symptoms under scrutiny. Johnstone and Crow (Crow 1980) based their distinction between type I and type II schizophrenia on the rating of just two symptoms in the eight-item Manchester Scale (Krawiecka et al. 1977). This is a short, efficient scale which is easy to use but may not be sufficiently comprehensive for studies with a strong emphasis on psychopathology. A number of other scales have been developed for rating negative symptoms including the Scale for the Assessment of Negative Symptoms (SANS) (Andreasen 1982), and the Present State Examination (PSE) versions 9 (Wing et al. 1974), and 10 (unpublished). However, the principles for rating negative symptoms are essentially the same as those for positive symptoms (Manchanda et al. 1989).

## 7.1 Problems for Studies in Chronic Patients

Any study of chronic patients has to take into account three particular issues which are not specifically considered in most acute studies. First, there is the problem of environmental over- and understimulation which has been thoroughly reviewed elsewhere (Hirsch 1986). Participation in a clinical trial may precipitate a relapse in stable quiescent chronic patients or, more likely, the stimulation and added interest of participating in the trial may itself lead to improvement, even of specifically schizophrenic symptoms. For example, McClelland and colleagues (1974) conducted a study to determine whether extrapyramidal side effects increase when anticholinergic medication is withdrawn from chronic patients on antipsychotic drugs. They found that more patients improved than deteriorated in both the placebo substituted group and the group maintained on their previous medication with respect to psychotic behaviours such as laughing, talking to themselves, posturing and mannerisms.

A second problem is that the patient may have been receiving excessive medication prior to entering the trial, producing side effects which have been interpreted as negative symptoms. For example, excessive sedation could lead to an appearance suggesting lack of drive or initiative, while parkinsonian side effects, including bradykinesia, could be misinterpreted as negative symptoms, such as flattening of affect or poverty of speech. A third problem is that the patients may not be responsive to any treatment, including both the old and new antipsychotic drugs. In such cases, demonstrating that a new putative antipsychotic is "as good as" an established drug could be misleading.

The design adopted by Kane et al. (1988) in their study of clozapine versus chlorpromazine in the treatment of refractory patients effectively dealt with many of these problems. After setting certain criteria to define failure to respond to existing medication, patients had time off from any medication. Improvement which occurred during this period could be ascribed to effective reduction in dosage and indicate excessive medication in the pretrial period. Patients were next treated with haloperidol 60 mg a day for 6 weeks as a standard high dose (but not megadose) treatment, in order to provide a common criterion of refractory to treatment. Patients who responded during this period were eliminated from the trial. Patients were then randomly allocated to receive chlorpromazine as required, up to 1800 mg a day, or clozapine up to 900 mg a day and the trial drug was given for 6 weeks. Significantly an improvement of 20% or more occurred in a significantly greater proportion of patients on clozapine as compared with those receiving chlorpromazine. This differential response indicated that the response to clozapine could not be due merely to environmental stimulation or both groups would have responded similarly, and indicated a specific response to clozapine as compared with chlorpromazine.

A more cautious design would have been to include a group administered placebo or low dose medication. Theoretically, if an experimental treatment gives the same result as a standard treatment it would not be possible to tell if the patient had responded beneficially to both treatments or failed to respond to either, thus inclusion of a placebo or very low dose treatment will overcome this problem.

For a further discussion of statistical issues, the effect of patient selection on outcome of clinical trials, the effect of social factors in determining the outcome of clinical trials, and a discussion of instruments available for rating clinical symptoms and social behaviour in clinical trials, the reader is referred to the recent text from the British Association of Psychopharmacology, *The Psycho pharmacology and Treatment of Schizophrenia* (Hirsch 1986).

## References

Andreasen NC (1982) Negative symptoms in schizophrenia: definition and reliability. Arch Gen Psychiatry 39:784–788

Creese R, Burt BR, Snyder FH (1976) Dopamine receptor binding predicts clinical and pharmacological potencies of antipsychotic drugs. Science 192:81–84

Crow TJ (1980) Molecular pathology of schizophrenia: more than one dimension of pathology? Br Med J 143:66–68

Curson DA, Hirsch SR, Platt SD, Bamber RW, Barnes TRE (1986) Does short term placebo treatment of chronic schizophrenia produce long term harm? Br Med J 293:726–728

Davis JM (1976) Comparative doses and costs of antipsychotic medication Arch Gen Psychiatry 33:858–861

Day SJ, Graham DF (1989) Sample size and power for comparing two or more treatment groups in clinical trials. Br Med J 299:663–665

Hirsch SR (1986) Influence of social experience and environment on the course of schizophrenia. In: Bradley PB, Hirsch SR (eds) The psychopharmacology and treatment of schizophrenia. Oxford University Press, Oxford

Hirsch SR, Macrae KD (1986) Essential elements in the design of clinical trials. In: Bradley PB, Hirsch SR (eds) The psychopharmacology and treatment of schizophrenia. Oxford University Press, Oxford

Hirsch SR, Gaind R, Rohde PD, Stevens BC, Wing JK (1973) Outpatient maintenance of chronic schizophrenic patients with long-acting fluphenazine: double-blind placebo trial. Br Med J i:633–637

Kane JM, Honigfeld G, Singer J, Meltzer H, The Clozaril Collaborative Study Group (1988) Clozapine for the treatment-resistant schizophrenic. Arch Gen Psychiatry 45:789–796

Krawiecka M, Goldberg D, Vaughan M (1977) A standardised psychiatric assessment scale for rating chronic psychotic patients. Acta Psych Scand 55:299–308

Manchanda R, Hirsch SR (1986) Does propranolol have an antipsychotic effect – a placebo-controlled trial in acute patients. Br J Psychiatry 148:701–707

Manchanda R, Hirsch SR, Barnes TRE (1989) A review of rating scales for measuring symptom changes in schizophrenia research. In: Thompson C (ed) The Instruments of Psychiatric Research. Wiley, Chichester

McClelland H, Blessed G, Bhate S, Ali N, Clarke PA (1974) The abrupt withdrawal of antiparkinsonian drugs in schizophrenic patients. Br J Psychiatry 124:151–159

Overall JE, Gorham DR (1962) The brief psychiatric rating scale. Psychol Rep 10:799–812

Seeman P, Lee T, Chang-Wong M, Wong K (1976) Antipsychotic drug doses and neuroleptic/dopamine receptors. Nature 261:717–719

Wing JK, Cooper JE, Sartorious N (1974) The Measurement and Classification of Psychiatric Symptoms. Cambridge University Press, Cambridge

# Evaluation of Drugs in Alzheimer's Disease and Age-Associated Memory Impairment

T.H. Crook, B.A. Johnson, and G.J. Larrabee[1]

A major issue in assessing the efficacy of drugs for late-life cognitive disorders is that of clinical relevance or "ecologic validity." It has been argued (Crook 1983; 1985a; Larrabee and Crook 1988; Leber 1986) that measures of treatment effects should bear a clear relationship to the behavioral problems for which treatment is undertaken. These behavioral problems may be assessed through rating scales completed by the clinician, the family of the patient, and sometimes the patient himself. Behavioral capacities may also be assessed directly through objective, psychometric performance tests. A major problem with most psychometric tests, however, is that they are abstract and bear little relationship to the behavioral problems for which drugs may be prescribed.

An effort was begun a decade ago to develop a battery of clinically relevant performance tests for assessing treatment effects in adult onset cognitive disorders. The first generation of tests was developed in collaboration with Drs. Steven Ferris, Charles Flicker, and other investigators (e.g., Ferris and Crook 1983; Crook 1985a; Ferris et al. 1986a). In 1985 we began an accelerated effort to develop a second generation of measures utilizing stage-of-the-art computer and laser-disk technology to closely simulate tasks of daily life on which performance is often impaired in adult-onset cognitive disorders.

Our objectives in test development were as follows:

1. To develop measures that relate closely to the behavioral problems for which treatment may be undertaken in adult-onset cognitive disorders.
2. To employ academically sound paradigms of human cognitive processes.
3. To develop measures sensitive to both normal age-related memory loss and cognitive symptoms seen early in the course of adult-onset cognitive disorders.
4. To develop measures that meet the highest standards of inter-rater and test-retest reliability.
5. To develop tests that are appropriate for different languages and cultures and, thus, appropriate for use in multinational drug trials.
6. To develop measures available in at least five alternate forms for repeated use in drug trials.

[1] Memory Assessment Clinics, Inc., 8311 Wisconsin Ave., Bethesda, MD 20814, USA

Methodology of the Evaluation of Psychotropic Drugs
Editors: O. Benkert, W. Maier, and K. Rickels
(Psychopharmacology Series 8)
© Springer-Verlag Berlin Heidelberg 1990

7. To develop extensive normative data in different cultures and extensive data on the patterns of deficits seen in different neurologic disorders.
8. To develop measures sensitive to drug effects including measures based on paradigms of learning and memory found sensitive to drug effects in experimental animals.
9. To develop a battery measuring empirically as well as theoretically distinct parameters of cognitive function.
10. To develop an assessment system in which relevant behavioral capacities are assessed through self-ratings, family ratings, and clinician ratings, as well as through performance tests.

In an effort to meet these objectives, research aimed at test development and refinement, as well as drug testing, was undertaken and is now under way in multiple clinics, universities, and community settings in Belgium, Denmark, England, Finland, France, Italy, Sweden, and the United States. In this paper we describe several of the tests in the battery and present data from several studies conducted in the United States. For a more general discussion of theoretical issues related to the assessment of drug effects and other tests that may be used in treatment evaluation studies, we refer the reader to two other recent papers (i.e., Flicker 1988; Larrabee and Crook 1988). A review of other computerized tests is provided by Maulucci and Eckhouse (1988).

## 1 Computerized Laser-Disk Performance Tests

### 1.1 Hardware and Software

Although our battery of performance tests is computerized, we believe strongly in using electronic technology to simulate clinical reality. Thus, in no case are subjects required to interact with the computer during testing. We do not employ keyboards, joysticks, or other manipulanda with which subjects are differentially familiar in testing. Rather, a tester operates the computer and laser-disk equipment and the subject responds either verbally, by touching a large touch-sensitive monitor to register a response, or by operating familiar manipulanda (e.g., a telephone) interfaced with the computer.

The equipment that constitutes a computerized test station is the same worldwide. Hardware is as follows:

- An American Telephone and Telegraph (AT&T) 6300 computer with a 20 megabyte hard disk drive.
- Installed in the computer is an Image Capture Board (ICB) produced by AT&T for presentation of computer generated graphics.
- A Pioneer LDV 6010 laser-disk player.
- A laser-disk produced by our organization and mastered by 3M Corporation. For each language in which we test.
- A Sony 19', 1910, color monitor with a touchscreen installed by our organization.

- A printer for simultaneous hard-copy as well as electronic storage of responses.
- Various computer-interfaced manipulanda and control devices developed by our organization.

All software for test administration and scoring, data storage, and data communication was written by one of the authors (B.A.J.) and his staff. The primary programming "language" in which the tests were written is "C." Assembly language is used on tests with strict hardware timing requirements.

## 1.2 Description of Tests

Following is a description of tests employed in studies of neurologically intact groups. The measures are employed in normative studies and in drug trials in persons with normal, age-related memory loss. The diagnostic term for this latter condition is Age-Associated Memory Impairment (AAMI; Crook et al. 1986a). Different versions of the test battery are employed in studies of Alzheimer's disease and other neurologic disorders. In drug development, tests are "tailored" to the disorder under study and to the neurochemical and behavioral profile of the drug under investigation.

### 1.2.1 Telephone Dialing (Without Interference)

This task is a variation on the standard digit-recall test and is intended to provide greater ecologic validity. An earlier, noncomputerized version of the test was validated in normal aging and AD and described a decade ago (Crook et al. 1980). In the current procedure subjects are shown series of 7- or 10-digit numbers (as in local or long distance American telephone numbers) on the monitor screen and asked to read the series aloud. Immediately after the final digit is read, the series disappears from the screen and subjects are instructed to dial the complete number on a push-button phone interfaced with the computer. A rotary dial phone is used in some European locations. Numbers dialed by the subject are automatically displayed on the screen as they are dialed, but no other feedback is provided. Eight trials are conducted, four at each of the two series lengths. In scoring, credit is given for each digit dialed in the correct position regardless of errors made elsewhere in the sequence.

### 1.2.2 Telephone Dialing (With Interference)

This task proceeds in the same manner as the dialing task described above, except that after subjects have completed dialing, they are presented with either a "busy" signal or the sound of a "ringing" telephone. If a busy signal occurs, the command "Please Redial" appears on the video screen, and subjects are then asked to redial the number. Scoring is the same as in the previous telephone dialing task.

### 1.2.3 Name-Face Association – Immediate Recall

This test is modeled on the most frequent behavioral problem involving memory, that is, forgetting the names of persons after introduction. An earlier, less realistic version of a test modeled on this problem was described several years ago (Ferris et al. 1986b). In the current test, subjects are shown live color video recordings (stored on laser-disk) of persons (actors) introducing themselves individually by common first names. After a series of introductions, recall is assessed by presenting the same persons in a different order and asking the subject to provide the name of each person. To provide the subject with expressive, acoustical, and other cues available in daily life, individuals who appear on the screen during the recall phase of the test indicate the city where they reside with the statement "I'm from ________." Following this statement, subjects are asked to provide the individual's name. In phase 1 of the test, subjects are shown three different series of introductions consisting of two, four, and six individuals, and recall occurs following each series. In phase 2, subjects are shown 14 individuals (in different sequences) in three consecutive trials to measure acquisition. Scoring is based on the total correct for each recall condition.

### 1.2.4 Name-Face Association – Delayed Recall

This phase of the test is administered approximately 40 min after the third acquisition trial described above. For a fourth time subjects are shown the 14 individuals introduced in the acquisition paradigm. No introductions are provided for the delayed recall trial; rather, the subjects' task is to recall the individual's name when presented with the "I'm from ________" portion of the video. Scoring is for total names correctly recalled.

### 1.2.5 Recognition of Faces – Signal Detection

This test of facial recognition employs an advanced version of a paradigm developed previously and validated in normal aging and AD (Ferris et al. 1980). Subjects are shown 156 actual facial photographs, each displayed on a touch-screen monitor for 2.6 s. The subjects' task is to touch a "YES" or "NO" box displayed in color on the screen to indicate whether they have or have not seen the photograph earlier in the test session. Fifty of the faces are shown twice; the remainder are shown only once. Of those shown twice, the interval between first and second presentation is varied systematically from 0 to 4 min. Signal detection methods are employed to control for differing response criteria among subjects and the statistic d' is calculated at each delay interval.

### 1.2.6 Recognition of Faces – Signal Detection, Delayed

This test is a delayed version of the test described above. Approximately 40 min after the initial recognition test, subjects are shown 20 photographs, 10 of which were shown (only once) in the earlier phase of the test and 10 of which are being shown for the first time. The subjects' task is to identify those faces which are repeated by pressing the appropriate box ("YES" or "NO") on the touchscreen and, again, signal detection methods are used in scoring.

### 1.2.7 Recognition of Faces – Delayed Nonmatching to Sample

This facial recognition task employs a paradigm found sensitive to the effects of aging and, the effects of drugs designed to improve cognition (Crook and Larrabee, Submitted for publication). On the first trial of this test, subjects are shown a single facial photograph on the touchscreen monitor and asked to touch the face. On each of 24 subsequent trials a "new" face is added to the array, and the subjects' task is to identify the new face by touching it on the monitor. Each trial is separated from the preceding trial by an 8-s interval, during which the screen is blank. Subjects receive feedback for their responses on each trial in the form of a red square that appears momentarily around the photograph if it is correctly identified. Two scores are computed. The first is the number correctly identified until subjects make their first error. The second is the total number correctly identified.

### 1.2.8 Reaction Time

This is a variation on a standard information-processing paradigm in which the task of driving a car and responding appropriately to changing traffic signals is simulated. On the screen subjects are shown a representation of a traffic light and representations of brake and accelerator pedals. Subjects are instructed to change pedals appropriately and as quickly as possible (using the dominant hand) when the light changes colors. The light changes at varying intervals of 3, 4, and 5 s, and both lift and travel time are recorded in milliseconds at each of these intervals.

### 1.2.9 Divided Attention

This test follows the same format as the reaction time measure previously described, but in addition to the driving task subjects are presented with simulated radio weather and traffic reports while performing the driving task. Subjects are asked to recall as much information as possible from the reports in a free-recall format. The number of facts correctly recalled in each of the two reports is scored.

### 1.2.10 Selective Reminding

This test follows the standard selective reminding paradigm using common grocery list items as the stimuli to be recalled. The test derives from a measure validated some years ago (McCarthy et al. 1981). On the first trial of the test, subjects are shown a list of 15 grocery items that are listed individually on the video screen. Immediately following presentation of the 15 items, subjects are asked to recall as many items as possible in any order. On subsequent trials, subjects are provided only with names of items not recalled on the previous trial, although recall of the entire list is requested. Thus, subjects are "selectively reminded" of the words they omitted on the previous trial. Scoring is for the following parameters of performance: total recall, summed across all five test trials; long-term storage or LTS (i.e., words that have been recalled at least once without reminding are assumed to remain in LTS on successive trials, even if the subject does not mention them subsequently); consistent long-term retrieval or CLTR (consistent recall of a word in LTS, to the end of the test trials); and half-hour delayed free recall. Scores for LTS and CLTR are cumulative over the five continuous learning trials. The test is terminated prior to five trials if the subject recalls the entire list on two successive trials.

### 1.2.11 First-Last Names

This is a test of associative learning and memory of verbal stimuli. On each of five trials, subjects are presented with a series of six paired first and last names, followed by a presentation of the last names only. The subjects' task is to recall the first name which was paired with each last name. As in Selective Reminding, the test extends to five trials unless a subject correctly recalls all the first names on two successive trials prior to the fifth trial. The score is the total of first names correctly identified for each trial.

### 1.2.12 Misplaced Objects

A simplified, noncomputerized version of this test was described some years ago (Crook et al. 1979). In the present computerized test, subjects are shown computer representations of 20 common objects that are frequently misplaced (e.g., eyeglasses) and the detailed interior of a 12-room house. During the first phase of the test the house remains displayed on the screen and subjects are asked to place each object, one at a time, in a location where it can later be recalled. The object is placed simply by touching the screen in the desired location, whereupon an accurate computer representation of the object appears in that location on the screen. The only limitation in object placement is that no more than two objects can be placed in a single room. After all objects are placed, the subject goes on to other tests. Approximately 40 min later, recall is tested. In this phase, the rooms are again displayed and the subjects' task is to recall the room in which each object was placed. They do so by touching the correct room and, if the response is correct, the object appears briefly in the room. Subjects are allowed two attempts to recall each object and the two attempts are scored separately. There are no time limits on either placement or recall of objects.

### 1.2.13 Narrative Recall

This test follows the design of older narrative recall tests in which subjects are required to recall the content of a paragraph read to them by the tester. In this case, however, subjects watch a 6-min television news broadcast. They are then given a series of 25 factual, multiple-choice questions on the touchscreen and asked to select the correct answer by touching a corresponding box on the screen. There are no time limits for response and the score is simply the number of correct responses.

### 1.2.14 Topographic Memory

Two tests of topographic memory are employed. In the first, subjects are shown a live video recording, from the driver's perspective, of an automobile traversing a circuitous route through a city. Immediately after viewing, the video is shown for a second time. However, on this occasion the car appears to stop at each intersection, arrows appear on the monitor, and subjects are asked to identify which way the car turned on the earlier "trip." The second topographic memory test employs a road map with international map symbols, rather than a live video recording. In this case, the entire map is shown on the screen, the computer traces increasingly complex routes, and the task of the subject is to retrace the routes on the touchscreen.

## 2 Sensitivity of Tests to the Effects of Age

In the past several years attention has focused on developing treatments for normal age-related memory loss (Crook and Larrabee 1988a; Crook 1989). The term adopted for this phenomenon by workgroups of the National Institute of Mental Health in the United States is Age-Associated Memory Impairment (AAMI; Crook et al. 1986a). Of course, measures of treatment effects in AAMI must be sensitive to the symptomatology of the condition, that is, to the memory loss that occurs in normal aging.

In an effort to establish the sensitivity of the test battery to the effects of normal aging, the measures have been administered to more than 3000 healthy normal subjects of different ages. Results for each test have been or will be reported in separate publications (e.g., Crook and West (in press); Crook et al. 1988; Crook and Larrabee 1988b), but in this report, results from several studies in the United States from three specific tests will be cited.

### 2.1 Name-Face Acquisition

Table 1 presents demographic data for a sample of 1547 healthy normal subjects to whom the test was administered in the United States. It is noteworthy that all subjects are well educated and, most important, that subjects in the older groups are actually superior to subjects in the youngest group on the Wechsler Adult Intelligence Scale (WAIS) Vocabulary Subtest – a standard index of verbal intelligence. Thus, any difference in memory test performance among age groups cannot reasonably be accounted for by differences in education or general intellectual function.

Table 2 presents results of test administration for the three acquisition trials and the delayed recall trial. These same results are shown graphically in Fig. 1. It

**Table 1.** Name-face association test, demographics

| Age group (*n*) | Gender (%F) | Age $\bar{X}$ | Age SD | Education $\bar{X}$ | Education SD | WAIS vocabulary $\bar{X}$ | WAIS vocabulary SD |
|---|---|---|---|---|---|---|---|
| 18–39 (328) | 53 | 26.00 | 7.33 | 14.78 | 2.19 | 58.43 | 10.09 |
| 40–49 (154) | 69 | 44.64 | 2.71 | 16.27 | 2.88 | 61.46 | 10.26 |
| 50–59 (428) | 65 | 54.64 | 2.88 | 16.09 | 2.70 | 62.96 | 9.70 |
| 60–69 (430) | 57 | 64.23 | 2.84 | 15.70 | 2.78 | 63.18 | 9.42 |
| 70+ (207) | 57 | 73.63 | 3.77 | 15.80 | 3.03 | 64.72 | 9.52 |

**Table 2.** Age group comparisons, name-face association test acquisition trials

| Age group (*n*) | 18–39 (328) | 40–49 (154) | 50–59 (428) | 60–69 (430) | 70+ (207) | Group Differences *F* value (sign of *F*) | Tukey *B* |
|---|---|---|---|---|---|---|---|
| $\bar{X}$ | 4.89 | 3.43 | 2.92 | 2.33 | 1.81 | 83.13 | 1–2,3,4,5 |
| 1st presentation of 14 | | | | | | | 2–3,4,5; 3–4,5 |
| SD | 2.89 | 2.35 | 2.33 | 1.77 | 1.76 | (0.0) | 4–5 |
| $\bar{X}$ | 10.08 | 8.05 | 7.08 | 6.11 | 4.80 | 106.33 | 1–2,3,4,5 |
| 2nd presentation of 14 | | | | | | | 2–3,4,5; 3–4,5 |
| SD | 3.25 | 3.28 | 3.33 | 3.15 | 3.21 | (0.0) | 4–5 |
| $\bar{X}$ | 12.39 | 10.56 | 9.86 | 8.57 | 6.72 | 108.66 | 1–2,3,4,5 |
| 3rd presentation of 14 | | | | | | | 2–4,5; 3–4,5 |
| SD | 2.47 | 3.18 | 3.38 | 3.67 | 3.70 | (0.0) | 4–5 |
| $\bar{X}$ | 12.20 | 10.16 | 9.19 | 8.04 | 6.13 | 114.36 | 1–2,3,4,5 |
| Delayed presentation of 14 | | | | | | | 2–3,4,5; 3–4,5 |
| SD | 2.78 | 3.45 | 3.58 | 3.77 | 3.76 | (0.0) | 4–5 |

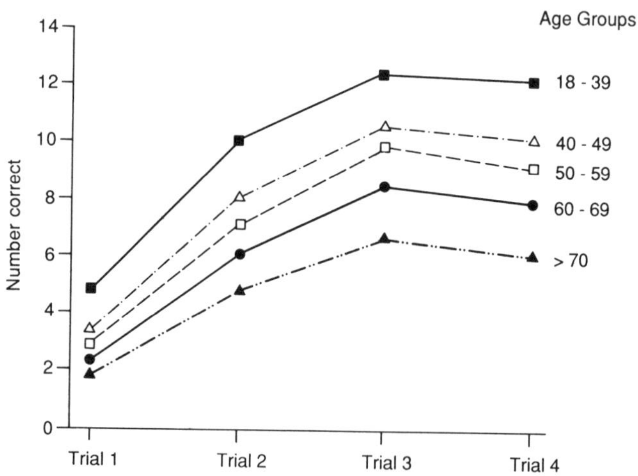


**Fig. 1.** Name-face association; acquisition trials

is clear from this data that a striking decade-by-decade decline in performance begins in mid-life and continues thereafter. Of course, in AAMI drug trials this deficit is a target of treatment.

## 2.2 Facial Recognition – Signal Detection Paradigm

Quite a different pattern of age-sensitivity is reflected in facial recognition as measured through a signal-detection paradigm. Demographic data for an American sample to whom the test was administered are presented in Table 3. Results of testing are presented in Table 4 and shown graphically in Fig. 2.

It is apparent from these data that the pattern of change in performance with age is quite different than on the Name-Face acquisition measure shown previously. It is only among persons 70 years and older that a reliable deficit is seen at many of the retention intervals. Beyond that observation, of particular im-

**Table 3.** Recognition of faces test, demographics

| Age group | Gender | Age | | Education | | WAIS vocabulary | |
|---|---|---|---|---|---|---|---|
| ($n$) | (%F) | $\bar{X}$ | SD | $\bar{X}$ | SD | $\bar{X}$ | SD |
| 18–39 (88) | 56 | 30.40 | 5.31 | 15.73 | 2.46 | 57.88 | 10.98 |
| 40–49 (68) | 74 | 44.85 | 2.83 | 16.00 | 2.72 | 60.60 | 10.66 |
| 50–59 (193) | 66 | 54.42 | 2.83 | 16.10 | 2.71 | 62.20 | 9.33 |
| 60–69 (189) | 67 | 64.53 | 2.75 | 15.55 | 2.81 | 62.10 | 9.69 |
| 70+ (95) | 63 | 73.43 | 3.58 | 15.80 | 3.02 | 62.15 | 10.92 |

**Table 4.** Age group comparisons recognition of faces

| Age group ($n$) | | 1<br>18–39<br>(88) | 2<br>40–49<br>(68) | 3<br>50–59<br>(193) | 4<br>60–69<br>(189) | 5<br>70+<br>(95) | $F$ value<br>(sign of F) | Tukey B |
|---|---|---|---|---|---|---|---|---|
| D'zero | Mean | 3.23 | 3.20 | 2.85 | 2.67 | 2.20 | 24.44 | 1,2–3,4,5; 3,4–5 |
| | SD | 0.69 | 1.09 | 0.75 | 0.81 | 0.85 | 0.00 | |
| D'one | Mean | 2.50 | 2.45 | 2.26 | 2.18 | 1.77 | 11.38 | 1–4,5; 2,3,4–5 |
| | SD | 0.79 | 1.14 | 0.75 | 0.77 | 0.79 | 0.00 | |
| D'two | Mean | 2.37 | 2.38 | 2.05 | 1.95 | 1.55 | 18.78 | 1,2–3,4,5; 3,4–5 |
| | SD | 0.77 | 1.06 | 0.72 | 0.62 | 0.69 | 0.00 | |
| D'three | Mean | 1.89 | 1.89 | 1.86 | 1.84 | 1.37 | 8.73 | 1,2,3,4–5 |
| | SD | 0.73 | 0.94 | 0.71 | 0.72 | 0.69 | 0.00 | |
| D'four | Mean | 1.42 | 1.31 | 1.27 | 1.28 | 1.02 | 5.46 | 1,2,3,4–5 |
| | SD | 0.69 | 0.58 | 0.58 | 0.62 | 0.53 | 0.00 | |
| D'forty | Mean | 1.15 | 1.38 | 1.11 | 0.96 | 0.65 | 11.29 | 2–4,5; 1,3,4–5 |
| | SD | 0.84 | 0.80 | 0.76 | 0.68 | 0.57 | 0.00 | |

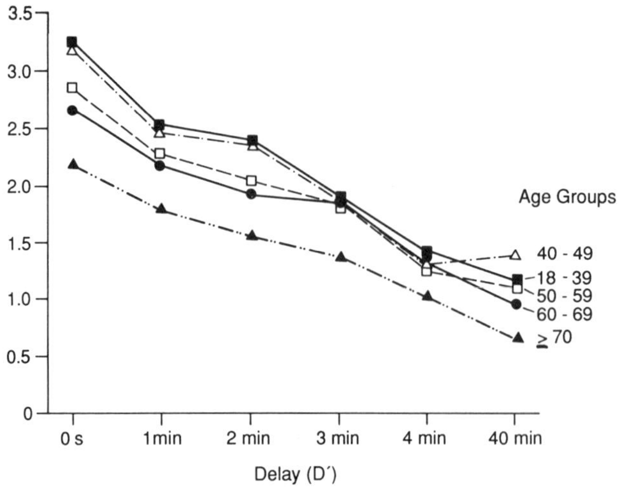


**Fig. 2.** Recognition of faces test

portance is the finding that the most reliable change with age seen in this measure is at the "zero second" retention interval. This is a measure of attention rather than memory and this attentional difference, as well as the deficit in acquisition shown previously on the Name-Face Test, may be an appropriate target for drug treatment in AAMI trials.

## 2.3 Telephone Dialing Test

The demographic characteristics of subjects in a study of the effects of age on the Telephone Dialing Test are shown in Table 5. Study results are shown in Table 6 and illustrated in Fig. 3. It is apparent from these data that a highly significant decline with age is seen at ten digits and this decline is exaggerated when the information must be retained and redialing must occur following a busy signal (the interference condition). Again, this age-related deficit may be seen as an appropriate target of drug treatment in AAMI.

**Table 5.** Telephone dialing with interference test, demographics

| Age group | Gender | Age | | Education | | Wais vocabulary | |
|---|---|---|---|---|---|---|---|
| (*n*) | (%F) | $\bar{X}$ | SD | $\bar{X}$ | SD | $\bar{X}$ | SD |
| 18–39 (244) | 52 | 24.67 | 7.34 | 14.43 | 1.98 | 58.83 | 9.85 |
| 40–49 (74) | 64 | 44.49 | 2.55 | 15.94 | 2.92 | 62.89 | 9.56 |
| 50–59 (197) | 62 | 54.88 | 2.97 | 16.29 | 2.72 | 64.31 | 9.56 |
| 60–69 (212) | 52 | 63.93 | 2.81 | 15.81 | 2.77 | 63.97 | 9.14 |
| 70+ (105) | 53 | 73.74 | 3.91 | 15.31 | 2.98 | 66.00 | 9.27 |

**Table 6.** Age group comparisons, telephone dialing test

| Age group (*n*) | 18–39 (244) | 40–49 (74) | 50–59 (197) | 60–69 (212) | 70+ (105) | Group Differences *F* value (sign of *F*) | Tukey B |
|---|---|---|---|---|---|---|---|
| $\bar{X}$ | 6.66 | 6.71 | 6.72 | 6.65 | 6.49 | 3.52 | 1–5 |
| Average 7 digits | | | | | | | 2–5 |
| before interference | | | | | | | 3–5 |
| SD | 0.56 | 0.40 | 0.45 | 0.51 | 0.72 | (.01) | 4–5 |
| $\bar{X}$ | 7.73 | 7.72 | 7.50 | 6.96 | 6.24 | 21.42 | 1–4,5 |
| Average 10 digits | | | | | | | 2–4,5 |
| before interference | | | | | | | 3–4,5 |
| SD | 1.49 | 1.51 | 1.57 | 1.64 | 1.58 | (0.0) | 4–5 |
| $\bar{X}$ | 6.15 | 6.02 | 5.91 | 5.64 | 5.07 | 16.88 | 1–4,5 |
| Average 7 digits | | | | | | | 2–5 |
| after interference | | | | | | | 3–5 |
| SD | 0.98 | 1.02 | 1.12 | 1.35 | 1.53 | (0.0) | 4–5 |
| $\bar{X}$ | 5.57 | 5.13 | 4.82 | 4.08 | 3.20 | 34.64 | 1–3,4,5 |
| Average 10 digits | | | | | | | 2–4,5 |
| after interference | | | | | | | 3–4,5 |
| SD | 2.00 | 2.05 | 1.90 | 1.89 | 1.84 | (0.0) | 4–5 |

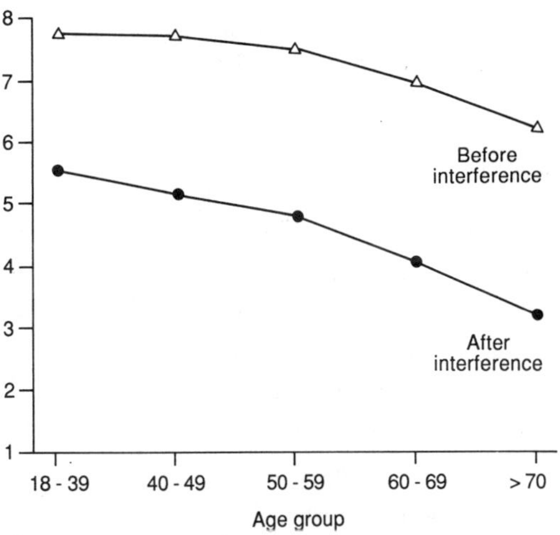


**Fig. 3.** Telephone dialing with interference; average ten digits

## 3 Relationships Among Tests

Factor analytic studies in different populations are described in detail elsewhere (Crook and Larrabee 1988b; Larrabee and Crook 1989). The results of a factor analytic study in a population of normal subjects are presented in Table 7 and results of a study in AAMI are presented in Table 8. It is apparent from these

**Table 7.** Varimax-rotated principal components analysis, immediate recall raw scores (from Crook and Larrabee 1988b)[a]

| Variables | Factors 1 | 2 | 3 | 4 |
|---|---|---|---|---|
| Name-face association, sum | 0.77 | | | |
| Name-face association, 6 faces | 0.50 | | | -0.59 |
| Narrative recall | 0.58 | 0.34 | | |
| Telephone dialing, 3 digits | | | | 0.81 |
| Telephone dialing, 10 digits | 0.55 | | | |
| Misplaced objects, first try | 0.61 | -0.54 | -0.32 | |
| Misplaced objects, second try | | 0.88 | | |
| Recognition of faces – signal detection | 0.61 | | | |
| Reaction time, lift component | | -0.49 | 0.52 | |
| Reaction time, travel component | | | 0.85 | |
| Recognition of faces – delayed nonmatching | 0.41 | | -0.40 | |

[a] Loadings of 0.30 or greater are reported; $n = 158$.

**Table 8.** Varimax-rotated principal components analysis, immediate recall without interference (from Larrabee and Crook, 1989)[a]

| Variables | Factors 1 | 2 | 3 | 4 |
|---|---|---|---|---|
| Name-face association, 6 faces | 0.66 | | | |
| Name-face association, sum | 0.83 | | | |
| Recognition of faces – delayed nonmatching | 0.30 | | | 0.64 |
| Recognition of faces – signal detection | | 0.32 | | 0.68 |
| Reaction time, lift component | | | 0.73 | -0.30 |
| Reaction time, travel component | | | 0.78 | |
| Telephone dialing, 7 digits | | 0.80 | | |
| Telephone dialing, 10 digits | | 0.80 | | |
| Incidental memory for traffic broadcast | 0.51 | 0.37 | | |
| First-last names | 0.72 | | | |
| Selective reminging – total CLTR | 0.71 | | | |

[a] Loadings of 0.30 or greater are reported; $n = 110$.

tables that the tests do indeed assess empirically as well as theoretically distinct parameters of cognitive functions in different populations. This allows for independent analysis of drug effects on distinct memory abilities.

## 4 Alternate Forms

As noted previously, five or more alternate forms are available for each test in each language. Tables 9, 10, and 11 present results of studies equating three American forms of the three tests on which age-sensitivity data were presented previously.

As shown in these tables, different forms of the tests are quite similar in level of difficulty.

**Table 9.** Form equivalency analysis, name-face association

| MAC variable | Form A Mean | SD | Form B Mean | SD | Form C Mean | SD | *F* value (sign) |
|---|---|---|---|---|---|---|---|
| | ($n$ = 51) | | ($n$ = 54) | | ($n$ = 58) | | |
| Presentation of 14 name-face pairs | | | | | | | |
| First trial | 3.55 | 1.75 | 3.48 | 2.04 | 3.55 | 1.92 | 0.02 (0.98) |
| Second trial | 8.36 | 2.54 | 8.00 | 3.52 | 8.41 | 3.17 | 0.23 (0.79) |
| Third trial | 10.00 | 3.35 | 10.48 | 3.05 | 10.72 | 2.97 | 0.29 (0.75) |
| Delay | 10.73 | 2.24 | 10.12 | 3.36 | 10.14 | 3.19 | 0.17 (0.84) |

**Table 10.** Form equivalency analysis, recognition of faces

| MAC variable | Form A Mean | SD | Form B Mean | SD | Form C Mean | SD | *F* value (sign) |
|---|---|---|---|---|---|---|---|
| | ($n$ = 53) | | ($n$ = 57) | | ($n$ = 55) | | |
| D′ - no delay | 2.68 | 0.80 | 2.65 | 0.79 | 2.59 | 0.81 | 0.15 (0.86) |
| D′ - 1 min delay | 2.15 | 0.72 | 2.10 | 0.83 | 2.29 | 0.80 | 0.88 (0.42) |
| D′ - 2 min delay | 1.81 | 0.74 | 1.87 | 0.80 | 1.97 | 0.78 | 0.56 (0.57) |
| D′ - 3 min delay | 1.78 | 0.83 | 1.53 | 0.83 | 1.49 | 0.64 | 1.19 (0.31) |
| D′ - 4 min delay | 1.24 | 0.59 | 1.21 | 0.67 | 1.36 | 0.64 | 0.81 (0.45) |

**Table 11.** Form equivalency analysis, telephone dialing with interference

| MAC variable | Form A Mean | A SD | B Mean | B SD | C Mean | C SD | *F* value (sign) |
|---|---|---|---|---|---|---|---|
| No interference | | | | | | | |
| Average 7 digits | 6.66 | 0.48 | 6.55 | 0.53 | 6.66 | 0.50 | 0.88 (0.41) |
| Average 10 digits | 7.40 | 1.29 | 7.16 | 1.38 | 7.39 | 1.50 | 0.57 (0.56) |
| Before interference | | | | | | | |
| Average 7 digits | 6.66 | 0.58 | 6.52 | 0.60 | 6.61 | 0.65 | 0.76 (0.47) |
| Average 10 digits | 7.61 | 1.38 | 7.37 | 1.41 | 7.28 | 1.51 | 0.83 (0.43) |
| After interference | | | | | | | |
| Average 7 digits | 5.98 | 1.01 | 5.61 | 1.23 | 5.86 | 1.29 | 1.45 (0.23) |
| Average 10 digits | 5.19 | 2.01 | 4.71 | 1.96 | 4.91 | 1.85 | 0.91 (0.40) |
| | | $n = 59$ | $n = 57$ | $n = 58$ | | | |

## 5 Relationship Between Computerized Tests and Rating Scales

In addition to the computerized tests of everyday memory abilities, rating scales were developed to measure those same abilities from the perspectives of patients, family members, and clinicians. The patient scale is entitled the Memory Assessment Clinics Self-Rating Scale, or MAC-S, the scale for family members is entitled the MAC-F and measures the same behaviors, and the scale for clinicians (primarily psychiatrists or psychologists) is referred to as the MAC-P. Studies are now under-way to examine the interrelationships among these measures in a variety of different normal and neurologically impaired populations. Factor analyses have been conducted on the MAC-S and multiple reliable measures of self-reported memory abilities have been identified (Crook and Larrabee, in press). One study conducted among normal subjects (Larrabee et al. 1989) suggests that the typically minimal relationships between self-reported memory abilities and direct measures of those abilities on performance tests can be improved somewhat when items are quite specific and when nonjudgemental phrasing is used, as is done on the MAC-S. Data are presented in Table 12.

As illustrated in Table 12, correlations between self-report measures and direct performance measures are significant in many cases, but remain low in general. We nevertheless view self-rating data as important in AAMI studies, equivalent family rating data as important in AD studies, and clinician ratings as important in all drug studies in late-life cognitive disorders. If evidence of drug efficacy can be developed from multiple sources, certainly the case for efficacy is strengthened beyond that when only psychometric tests or rating scales are

**Table 12.** Principal components analysis of self-rated and immediate recall memory test scores

| | Factors | | | | |
|---|---|---|---|---|---|
| Variables | 1 | 2 | 3 | 4 | 5 |
| MAC-S ability | | | | | |
| Remote | 0.38 | 0.52 | | 0.47 | |
| Numeric | 0.41 | 0.33 | 0.41 | | |
| Everyday | 0.79 | | | | |
| Semantic | | 0.67 | | | |
| Spatial | | 0.61 | | | |
| MAC-S frequency | | | | | |
| Semantic | 0.65 | | 0.36 | | |
| Concentration | 0.43 | 0.66 | | | |
| Everyday | 0.79 | | | | |
| Forgetful | 0.83 | | | | |
| Facial | 0.63 | | | | –0.36 |
| Global speed of recall[a] | | | 0.76 | | |
| Global concern/distress[b] | 0.51 | 0.30 | 0.58 | | |
| GDS[c] | –0.56 | | | | |
| Computerized tests | | | | | |
| General | | 0.69 | | | |
| Attention/vigilance | | | | | 0.87 |
| Psychomotor speed | | | | 0.86 | |
| Attention | | | –0.60 | | |

[a] Global speed of recall: "Compared to the best your memory has ever been, how would you describe the speed with which you now remember things?"
[b] Global concern/distress: "How much concern or distress do you feel about your memory at this time?"
[c] GDS, Geriatric Depression Scale.
Performance factors are from Crook and Larrabee (1988b); $n = 125$. Loadings of 0.30 or higher are reported.

employed as outcome measures (Leber 1986). However, in the absence of data on performance tests, data from rating scales may not provide adequate evidence of efficacy to meet American and other drug regulatory standards.

## 6 Applications of Tests in Drug Trials

A major goal of test development has been standardization of methodology so that results obtained by different investigators and in different countries will be comparable. If this can be accomplished in drug trials, data may be pooled internationally for the purpose of examining efficacy and gaining permission from regulatory authorities to bring drugs for learning and memory to the marketplace.

Of course, such a lofty goal requires not only standardization of assessment techniques, but also agreement among investigators on fundamental issues related to the assessment of drug effects in late-life cognitive disorders. Among the issues of major significance are the following:

### 6.1 Are Placebo-Controlled Trials Necessary?

The answer to this question according to a developing consensus of international opinion is clearly yes. In the United States this consensus recommendation was made formally by an expert group convened by the Food and Drug Administration in June of 1989. It was recognized that patients with AAMI, early AD, and other late-life cognitive disorders are often capable of both subjective and objective improvement in the absence of treatment with an active compound in clinical trials. The placebo-response effect may be even more apparent among family members of the AD patient who are desperate for an effective treatment. Behavior of the patient in clinical trials may be carefully monitored and behavior that would otherwise go unnoticed may be taken as evidence of drug efficacy. Of course, objective tests will limit this phenomenon, but they are not immune from placebo effects.

### 6.2 Length of Treatment

Questions frequently arise among investigators or pharmaceutical companies sponsoring clinical trials concerning the optimal length of the trial to be undertaken. The answer to this question, of course, depends upon the effects of the drug and the goals of therapy. A single dip of a single person in a true Fountain of Youth would be sufficient to produce the desired effects and demonstrate efficacy beyond question. By contrast, a compound that slightly altered the course of a slowly and variably progressive disorder such as AD would likely require years of study in hundreds or thousands of patients. Studies designed to demonstrate that drugs alter the course of a normal developmental condition such as AAMI would require decades and would be impossible for all practical purposes.

At present we may assume that the goal of therapy is to produce acute improvement, to mitigate symptoms, rather than to alter the course of illness, and that the effect of a desirable drug must be apparent in no more than 3 to 6 months. Thus, the treatment duration in most trials will be 12 to 24 weeks. Trials with substances such as cholinesterase inhibitors that produce immediate effects may be shorter in duration, but the question of whether immediate effects are sustained must be addressed if a drug is to be clinically useful.

### 6.3 Magnitude of Treatment Effects

What is the magnitude of effect sufficient to declare that a drug is clinically useful in treating AD or AAMI? From a regulatory perspective, the answer to this question may vary from country to country. In the United States the standard of evidence necessary for regulatory approval is clear, that is the compound must exert clinically meaningful effects that are statistically different from the control substances with which it is compared (in this case placebo; Leber 1986). Of course, at issue in most cases will be the risk/benefit ratio of a drug. It is clear that drugs for treating AAMI must be quite safe (Crook 1986) and if this is the case, the magnitude effect may be quite small. By contrast, drugs with relatively serious side effects may be tolerable in AD, particularly if the magnitude of the effect is large.

It is important to emphasize that no drug has conclusively been shown to improve learning and memory and neither scientists, physicians, nor the public should expect miraculous effect from the first such compounds to be developed. In the absence of a conceptual breakthrough, it is likely that the clinical effects of the first generation of memory enhancing drugs will be modest and progress thereafter will be incremental. If we reject compounds with modest but reliable effects and await extraordinary compounds we will do no service to the scientific enterprise or to those persons for whom even a small effect is of immense significance.

## 7 Conclusions

In examining our objectives in test development and assessing progress to date we may draw the following conclusions:

1. Our battery of tests employing computer and laser-disk technology closely simulates many of the behavioral tasks of daily life on which performance is impaired in AAMI and on which such impairment is further exaggerated in AD and related neurologic disorders.
2. The paradigms on which the tests are based range from standard acquisition and recognition paradigms to more recently developed experimental paradigms such as delayed non-matching-to-sample.
3. The sensitivity of measures to normal age-related deficits and early Alzheimer's disease has been demonstrated. Novel neuroepidemiologic studies are now under way as well, using a mobile memory assessment center to gather normal population data. Additional studies are under way to characterize the pattern of cognitive deficits seen in neurologic disorders such as Parkinson's disease, stroke, head injury, AIDS dementia, and multiple sclerosis. Experiments are also under way to assess the effect of neurosurgical procedures on test performance.
4. Multiple reliability studies are under way and substantial technical data on both interrater and test-retest reliability are available from the authors.
5. The test battery with live video recording has been developed for and is now in use in multicenter drug trials in the following countries: Belgium, Canada, Denmark, England, Finland, France, Italy, Sweden, and the United States. Development is under way for Dutch, German, Spanish, Russian, and Japanese test batteries as well.

6. At least five alternate forms were developed for each test in each language and development will continue to ensure equivalency of all forms.
7. The normative data base now includes nearly 4000 persons, but development will continue toward a goal of an international normative data base in excess of 50,000 persons. As noted, descriptive studies in multiple neurologic disorders are under way.
8. Many of the tests are modeled on paradigms found sensitive to drug effects in experimental animals. Studies with experimental drugs designed to enhance cognition are now under way worldwide with more than a dozen compounds. Studies with experimental compounds such as scopolamine demonstrate that test performance is sensitive to experimentally induced neurochemical deficits.
9. Factor analytic studies suggest that the test battery assesses empirically, as well as theoretically, distinct parameters of cognitive functioning.
10. Data on drug effects are collected from rating scales as well as on computerized tests. Psychometrically sound scales have been developed and multiple studies are under way to examine interrelationships among test performance and ratings completed by patients, family members, and clinicians.

In summary, it may be argued that substantial progress has been made in developing sensitive and clinically relevant methods for assessing drug effects in late-life cognitive disorders. Parallel developments in drug development have provided a generation of new compounds for clinical evaluation. In view of this progress in both clinical assessment methodology and the synthesis of new compounds, it may be argued that we have reached the time when we may plan rather than dream of developing effective drugs for treating cognitive disorders of later life.

## References

Crook T (1983) Psychometric assessment in Alzheimer's disease. In: Reisberg B (ed) Alzheimer's disease: the standard reference book. Free Press, New York

Crook T (1985a) Cognitive assessment in the year 2000. In: Gaitz C, Niederehe G, Wilson N (eds) Aging 2000 our health care destiny: psychosocial issues. Springer-Verlag, New York

Crook T (1985b) Methods for evaluating psychotherapeutic drugs: psychoses associated with old-age. In: McMahon FG (ed) Principles and techniques of human research and therapeutics. Futura, Mount Kisco, NY

Crook T (1986) Drug effects in Alzheimer's disease. In: Brink TL (ed) Clinical gerontologist: a guide to assessment and interventions. Haworth, New York

Crook T (1989) Diagnosis and treatment of normal and pathologic memory impairment in later life. Semin Neurol 9:20–30

Crook T, Larrabee G (1988a) Age-associated memory impairment: diagnostic criteria and therapeutic strategies. Psychopharmacol Bull 24(4):509–514

Crook T, Larrabee G (1988b) Interrelationships among everyday memory tests: stability of factor structure with age. Neuropsychology 2:1–12

Crook T, Larrabee GJ (1989) Two procedures for evaluating facial recognition memory across the adult age span. (submitted)

Crook T, Larrabee GJ (in press) A self-rating scale for evaluating memory in everyday life. Psychol Aging

Crook TH, West RL (in press) Name recall performance across the adult life span. British Journal of Psychology

Crook T, Ferris S, McCarthy M (1979) The misplaced objects task: a brief test for memory dysfunction in the aged. J Am Geriatrics Soc 27:284–287

Crook T, Ferris S, McCarthy M (1980) Utility of digit recall tasks for assessing memory in the aged. J Consult Clin Psychol 48:228–233

Crook T, Bartus R, Ferris S, Whitehouse P, Cohen G, Gershon S (1986a) Age-associated memory impairment: proposed diagnostic criteria and measures of clinical change. Development Neuropsychol 2:261–276

Crook T, Salama M, Gobert J (1986b) A computerized test battery for detecting and assessing memory disorders. In: Bes A, Cahn J, Hoyer S, Marc-Vergnes JP, Wisniewski HM (eds) Senile dementias: early detection. John Libbey, London-Paris

Crook T, Johnson B, Youniss E, Kelly A, Zadeik A, Bahar H (1988) Behavioral consequences of normal cerebral aging. In: Maloine SA (ed) L'Vieillisement Cerebral Normal et Pathologique. Foundation Nationale de Gerontologie, Paris, pp 11–21

Ferris S, Crook T (1983) Cognitive assessment in mild to moderately severe dementia. In: Crook T, Ferris S, Bartus R (eds) Assessment in geriatric psychopharmacology. Mark Powley, New Canaan CT

Ferris S, Crook T, Clark E, McCarthy M (1980) Facial recognition memory deficits in normal aging and senile dementia. J Gerontol 35:707–741

Ferris S, Crook T, Bartus R, Flicker C (1986a) Assessing treatment effects: psychometric performance tests. In: Poon L, Crook T, Davis K, Eisdorfer C, Gurland B, Kaszniak A, Thompson L (eds) Handbook for clinical memory assessment of older adults. American Psychological Association, Washington, DC

Ferris S, Crook T, Flicker C, Reisberg B, Bartus R (1986b) Psychometric assessment of treatment effects. In: Poon L, Crook T, Davis K, Eisdorfer C, Gurland B, Kaszniak A, Thompson L (eds) Handbook for clinical memory assessment of older adults. American Psychological Association, Washington, DC

Flicker C (1988) Neuropsychological evaluation of treatment effects in the elderly: a critique of tests in current use. Psychopharmacol Bull 24(4):535–556

Larrabee GJ, Crook T (1988) Assessment of drug effects in age-related memory disorders: clinical, theoretical, and psychometric considerations. Psychopharmacol Bull 24(4):515–522

Larrabee GJ, Crook T (1989) Dimensions of everyday memory in age-associated memory impairment. Psychol Assess J Consult Clin Psychol 1:92–97

Larrabee GJ, West RL, Crook TH (1989) The association of memory complaint with everyday memory performance. Paper presented at the 17th Annual Meeting of the International Neuropsychological Society, Vancouver, BC, Canada

Leber P (1986) Establishing the efficacy of drugs with psychogeriatric indications. In: Crook T, Bartus R, Ferris S, Gershon S (eds) Treatment development strategies for Alzheimer's disease, Mark Powley, Madison, CT, pp 1–14

Maulucci RA, Eckhouse RH (1988) The use of computers in the assessment and treatment of cognitive disabilities in the elderly: a survey. Psychopharmacol Bull 24(4):557–564

McCarthy M, Ferris S, Clark E, Crook T (1981) Acquisition and retention of categorized material in normal aging and senile dementia. Exp Aging Res 7:127–135

# Testing the Efficacy of New Hypnotic Drugs

F. HOHAGEN and M. BERGER[1]

## 1 Introduction

Sleep disorders are a major concern in the field of health politics. Epidemiological studies have revealed that 25%-35% of the population suffers from insomnia and 12.5% demonstrate insomnia severe enough to warrant medical help (Lugaresi et al. 1987; Bixler et al. 1979). This indicates the urgency of developing adequate methods of treatment. Benzodiazepines prevail in current insomnia therapy because of their relatively safe and prompt sleep-inducing properties (Woods et al. 1987; Lohse Mūller-Oerlinghausen 1988). However, as knowledge of the total efficacy/side-effect spectrum of this group of drugs accumulates, the attitude towards them has become increasingly critical and reserved. The major problem aside from possible tolerance and thereby the potential for addiction (Tryer 1988) is the generation of rebound insomnia. This can occur in extended intake and can endure for several weeks after withdrawal of the drug (Kales et al. 1983). The sleeplessness which arises in conjunction with the discontinuation of benzodiazepine therapy may lead to the patient's continued demand for these substances since he is convinced that without them he will not be able to sleep at all. The extent of the problem is visible in the practical work with insomniac patients, a great number of whom were or are currently dependent on some type of benzodiazepine.

These considerations have led to a refined judgement of the quality of hypnotics. That means the drugs are no longer merely evaluated in regard to their immediate hypnotic effects, but also regarding their long-term effects and the prospect of tolerance levels and rebound insomnia. These new aspects have considerably stimulated studies in the area of hypnotics prompting the testing of medicaments already on the market and the search for novel substances, which show no tolerance, have a long-term effect, and are not tainted with the risk of rebound insomnia.

## 2 Legal Requirements by Drug Licencing Authorities

Generally speaking, the same licencing regulations as for all other medicaments apply to new hypnotic drugs. The licencing agencies require a new therapy to be

[1] Zentralinstitut für Seelische Gesundheit, J5, 6800 Mannheim, FRG

Methodology of the Evaluation of Psychotropic Drugs
Editors: O. Benkert, W. Maier, and K. Rickels
(Psychopharmacology Series 8)
© Springer-Verlag Berlin Heidelberg 1990

both safe and effective. The clinical efficacy of a substance can be tested in controlled studies, either against a placebo or against an already introduced and acknowledged standard drug. Each country is bound by its own specific legal regulations governing the proper conduction of clinical tests. Requirements for members of the European Community have been standardized and published (EEC 1987) FDA requirements apply in the U.S.A.

## 3 Methods

The basic problem of a study with hypnotics is how to record the target syndrome, the disturbed sleep. For one thing, the investigation has to rely on the subjective complaints of the patient. In order to evaluate the course of treatment and thus the efficacy of a hypnotic drug, the patient's statements must be standardized. Sleep quality questionnaires, PISQI (Pittsburgh Sleep Quality Index) (Buysee et al. 1988), sleep disorder intensity scales, and visual analog scales (Ott et al. 1985), are recommended instruments for quantifying patients' complaints. Daytime impairment should be assessed on the subjective level by adjective mood scales (von Zerssen 1986). Patients should keep a sleep log during the course of the study, which should also include dream reports. On the objective level sleep is diagrammed by polygraphic registration. EEG is recorded by two channels in positions C3 and C4, two channels for ocular movements (EOG), and two EMG channels for submental muscle tone. With these parameters sleep is divided according to the criteria of Rechtschaffen and Kales (1968) into four non-REM stages and one REM-sleep stage. In recent years increased use has been made of computer-aided analyses of frequency such as the fast Fourier transformation analysis. This may pave the way for new vistas in the field of pharmaceutical research, particularly research on hypnotic drugs. In addition ECG can be recorded and, depending on the problem, thoracal, abdominal, and nasal respiration, $PO_2$-, $PCO_2$-, and $O_2$ saturation, as well as tibialis-anterior electrodes and body temperature. A detailed description of polygraphic sleep registration can be found in the pertinent literature (McGregor et al. 1985; Guilleminault 1982).

Upon commencement of a polygraphic sleep investigation in a sleep laboratory, an adaptation night should be conducted. This appears necessary since sleep characteristics, even of a healthy proband, change during the first night, showing signs of insomnia. Subsequently, two baseline nights should be recorded since the intraindividual variability between two nights can be substantial (Webb and Campbell 1979; Brownman and Cartwright 1980).

With the technical development of mobile EEG units, polygraphic sleep recording is now possible beyond the confines of a conventional sleep laboratory. By means of a portable, mobile long-term EEG (Ives and Woods 1975) that records the biosignals via a small cassette recorder, studies of hypnotic drugs in the familiar home environment of the patient are now possible. The electrodes can be attached to the patient in the evening in his home and the cassette be picked up the following morning. Polygraphic sleep registration in the familiar home environment precludes the artificial situation in a sleep laboratory and might yield more realistic results. Other experimental techniques can be considered as alternatives to the mobile long-term EEG, for example, the telemetric (Kamp 1984) or telephonic (van der Weide and Kamp 1984) EEG transport from the patient's home into the sleep laboratory. The telephonic transport of biosignals is being used in several research groups in the U.S.A., while in European countries use of this method is subject to legal and financial limitations.

Though the artificial atmosphere in a sleep laboratory can produce adaptation difficulties, it can also improve the quality of sleep. In clinical work with insomniac patients it happens that patients convincingly and comprehensibly complain of insomnia, while the sleep polygram yields a regular sleep profile and the patient himself reports the following morning never having slept so well as during the night in the sleep laboratory (de la Pena 1977). This phenomenon may be the consequence of a "paradoxical" intention – the patient tries hard to demonstrate his sleep disturbance, is thus no longer under pressure of the desire to sleep soundly, and as a result, can for the first time really sleep soundly again (demonstration effect). Mobile registration techniques such as the mobile long-term EEG might reduce the chances of such artifacts occurring in the much more artificial atmosphere of the sleep laboratory (Coates et al. 1981).

The excessive daytime fatigue of many insomniac patients can be ameliorated as sleep normalizes, thus serving as an indirect index of efficacy of a hypnotic drug. On the other hand, vigilance can be impaired during the day by hypnotic drugs whose half-life is long. The Multiple Sleep Latency Test (Westbrook and Keeman 1986), the Multiple Maintenance of Wakefulness Test (Mittler et al. 1982), and the Vienna Vigilance Test (Meyer-Evert and Wismans 1984), all of which are described in detail in the literature, are effective instruments for assessing vigilance. Besides these methods, others such as measuring saccadic eye movements (Hofferberth 1986) and pupillography (Yoss et al. 1970; Schmidt and Fortin 1982) are also employed. Psychometric tests seem to be necessary, especially when testing hypnotic drugs with a long half-life since these drugs can impaire cognitive and mnesic functions.

## 4 Selection of Patients

In compiling groups of patients various requirements must be met. First it has to be considered that sleep characteristics are not constant, that their quality and quantity change in the course of a lifetime (Williams et al. 1974). While a young person generally sleeps 7–8 h, an older person needs only 5–6 h of sleep. Compared with the sleep of a young person, the sleep of the elderly is more "superficial," i.e., the delta sleep segment (stages 3 and 4 according to Rechtschaffen and Kales) shrinks considerably, and the sleep polygram is interrupted by more frequent waking phases. The REM latency, meaning the time between sleep onset and the appearance of the first REM phase, becomes more variable with age. Sleep latency increases, sleep efficacy and total duration of sleep both decrease. These changes must be considered when evaluating sleep.

In planning studies, it is of the utmost importance that patient groups be comparable in age so that usable results can be achieved.

Gender-specific differences must also be considered in planning and evaluating studies of hypnotic drugs. Elderly men sleep worse than elderly women, while women subjectively suffer more from their sleep disorders, thereby complaining more frequently about them than do their male counterparts (Spiegel 1981). This phenomenon must also be taken into account when evaluating subjective statements.

As for all studies involving psychopharmacological drugs, the rule applies that patients must be free of medication acting on the central nervous system. It is well known that not only psychopharmaca but all other drugs with central nervous effects can alter the sleep EEG. Important in this connection are among others beta blockers, gyrase inhibitors, or hormone preparations. With regard to psychotropic drugs, one must note that antidepressants suppress REM sleep (Chen 1979) and some MAO inhibitors additionally decrease the delta sleep segments (Steiger et al. 1987). Benzodiazepines also suppress the slow components of sleep and lead to an increase in the rapid frequencies (Borbély 1986a), whereby the half-life of these substances and their active metabolites must be considered.

If hypnotic drugs such as benzodiazepines are taken over a long period, rebound insomnia can occur when they are discontinued. In some cases the insomnia can last several weeks until the quality of sleep attains the level prior to medication. Following intake of benzodiazepines with a shorter half-life, a single dose can be enough to trigger rebound insomnia in the following drug-free night (Borbély 1986b). One must also find out whether the patient really suffers from primary insomnia or from insomnia induced by medication, signaling the development of tolerance and addiction. In this case, an insomnia study would be confounded by the problem of insomnia resulting from (discontinued) medication. Additionally, further vegetative and psychopathological withdrawal symptoms affecting sleep can appear after long-term intake of benzodiazepines and barbiturates. For this reason a minimum drug-free period of at least 4 weeks is advisable. This precludes any interference of such phenomena in the experiment, which would disturb results. It must be critically remarked, however, that particularly in conjunction with chronic intake of hypnotic drugs such as benzodiazepines with long-term efficacy, rebound insomnia eventually can persist even longer than 4 weeks.

Basically the same exclusion criteria apply to studies of hypnotic drugs as to most drug studies:

1. Therapy with a psychoactive preparation within the last 2 weeks. If hypnotics with a very long half-life were taken over a long time span a 4-week wash out period seems to be necessary.
2. Alcoholism and drug abuse.
3. Therapy with other medicaments, which could interfere pharmacodynamically.
4. Accompanying neuropsychiatric illness.

5. Any kind of severe illness, especially gastroenteric diseases or disturbed hepatic or renal function which might interfere with the resorption, metabolism, or excretion of the test substance.
6. Blood pressure above 150/90 or below 90/60 mm Hg.
7. Cardiovascular illness.
8. Clinically relevant, abnormal laboratory findings or other additional findings such as pathological ECG, EEG, or CT.

## 5 Diagnosis

To guarantee the comparability of studies, diagnoses should be made according to firmly defined, operationalized criteria. The DSM-III-R (APA 1987) provides such diagnostic criteria. For the diagnosis of "insomnia" the following criteria must be fulfilled:

1. The predominant complaint is one of difficulty in initiating or maintaining sleep, or of nonrestorative sleep (sleep that is apparently adequate in amount, but leaves the person feeling unrested).
2. The disturbance in (1) occurs at least three times a week for at least 1 month and is sufficiently severe to result in either a complaint of significant daytime fatigue or the observation by others of some symptom that is attributable to the sleep disturbance, e.g., irritability or impaired daytime functioning.
3. Occurrence not exclusively during the course of sleep-wake-schedule disorder or a parasomnia.

The DSM-III-R distinguishes further between insomnia as a consequence of another mental disorder, insomnia as a consequence of a known organic factor, and primary insomnia. Patients who are to be included in studies of hypnotic drugs should fulfill the diagnostic criterion "primary insomnia" according to the DSM-III-R. One can arrive at a DSM-III-R diagnosis by an unstructured interview or with the aid of the structured clinical interview for DSM-III-R (Spitzer et al. 1986). The SCID enables a standardized diagnosis, thereby improving diagnostic reliability. An additional section for the diagnostic category "Sleep Disorders" according to the criteria of the DSM-III-R has been developed by our group (Schramm et al. 1989).

In addition to the DSM-III-R criteria the classification according to the "Association of SleepDisorder Centers" (1979) is recommended.

The DSM-III-R considers only the subjective remarks of the patients for the diagnostic process. If possible, objective parameters of sleep quality should be used additionally to validate the statements. Polygraphic sleep recordings, as described initially, ensure an objective assessment of sleep. Their importance lies, among other things, in their capability of detecting and ruling out disorders such as nocturnal myoclonia or disorders of breathing regulation as cause of the subjective complaints about disturbed sleep (ASDC 1979). Furthermore, the polygraphic registration of sleep delivers objective data that provide information on the efficacy of a hypnotic drug. Insomnia is characterized in the sleep EEG by long latency of falling asleep, low sleep efficacy with shorter duration of sleep, frequent awakening with an overall fractioned sleep profile, as well as by frequently changing sleep stages and very little or a complete lack of delta sleep (Fig. 1).

It is a frequent phenomenon, however, that complaints of the patient and objective sleep laboratory data are divergent. Insomnia patients evaluate quality and duration of sleep often more negatively than these were assessed in the sleep laboratory, while the length of the falling asleep period is frequently overestimated (Frankel et al. 1976; Carskadon et al. 1976). It ought to be considered whether only those patients should be included in studies of hypnotic drugs whose polygraphic registration also demonstrates insomnia. The numerous problems of so-called pseudoinsomnia, in which a subjective impairment of sleep occurs in tandem with a normal sleep polygram, are currently subject to controversial discussion and have not yet been finally resolved (Trinder 1988).

In any case patients should be excluded from studies of hypnotic drugs whose insomnia results from ignoring the most important basic rules of sleep hygiene. Many patients complain of difficulties in falling asleep and maintaining sleep when they retire already at 9 p.m. and remain in bed until 8 a.m. Especially among older patients unrealistic expectations persist concerning the duration and quality of sleep. When the time in bed constitutes 11 h, sleep must almost inevitably be fractioned and may no longer be experienced as restorative. In selecting patients, it should also be considered whether the consumption of stimulating beverages such as colas, coffee, etc. might be the cause of the sleep disorder (Karacan et al. 1976; Bonnet et al. 1979). Nicotine, another CNS stimulant, is often overlooked. Heavy smokers seem to sleep more poorly than nonsmokers (Soldatos et al. 1980). Of course, insomnia due to environmental causes such as street noise, a snoring bed partner, etc., should not be treated with hypnotic drugs but by altering the disturbing circumstances. It goes without saying that patients must also abstain from psychostimulants such as appetite suppressors, which are also a frequent cause of sleep disorder.

## 6 Study Design

The efficacy of a hypnotic drug can be assessed and evaluated by the following methods. On the subjective level sleep quality questionnaires, adjective mood scales, visual analog scales, and intensity scales can quantify the complaints of the patients. On the objective level the MSLT, MWT, Vienna Vigilance Test, and other methods assess the daytime fatigue, while the polygraphic sleep recording in the sleep laboratory registers the patient's sleep. During the study the side effects are protocolled correspondingly or are recorded on a checklist of side effects and quantified as needed. Impairment of cognitive and mnesic functions can be tested with psychometric tests. The patients are informed as to the study and declare their written consent to participate.

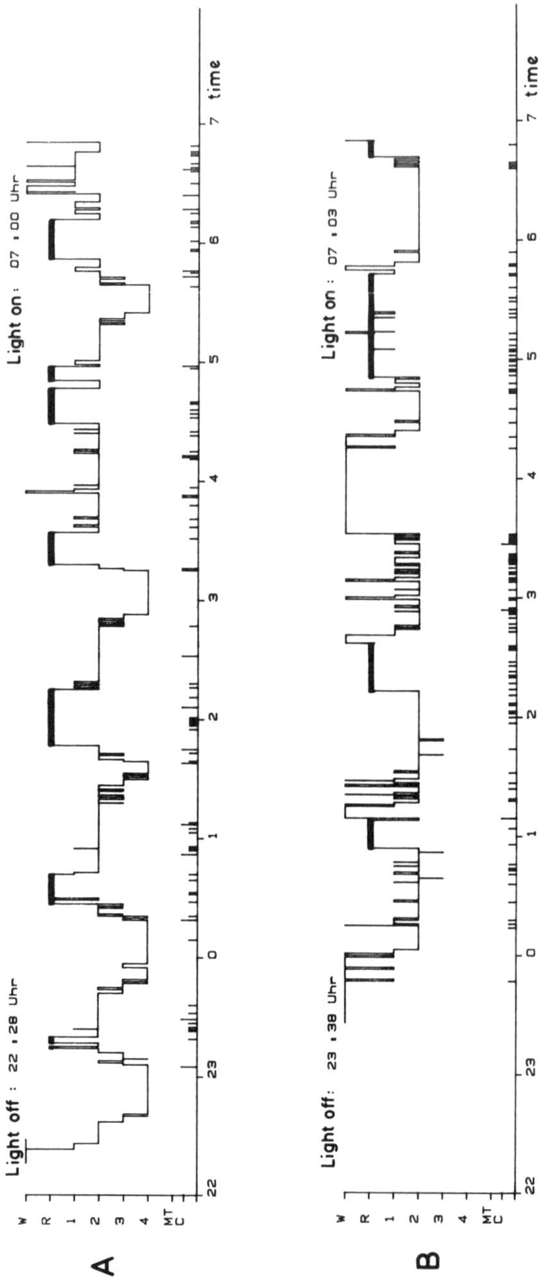


**Fig. 1.** **A** Normal sleep pattern of a young female adult. **B** Sleep pattern of an insomniac patient

Prior to the study the criteria of the efficacy of the hypnotic drug must be established. One source of information about the hypnotic effect is the subjective statement of the patient. Subjective sleep quality and impaired daytime functioning are quantified by the corresponding instruments. When the study design foresees a dose increase in the case of unsatisfactory therapy, a response criterion should be set in advance. If no such improvement occurs, the dose should be increased as fixed in the protocol beforehand.

Among the objective methods an improvement on the vigilance tests and a shortening of sleep latency, as well as a restoration of the physiological sleep profile with an increase in total delta sleep and an amelioration of sleep efficacy indicate the pharmacological effect of a hypnotic drug. If objective measurements have been obtained, they should also be considered for the decision whether a dose increase during the study because of insufficient response should take place.

As with all medicament studies, trials of hypnotic drugs should strive for double-blind conditions. This is, however, linked with the problem that patients might notice administration of the drug because of certain side effects (sedation, dry mouth, etc.). The possibility of administering an active placebo such as methylscopolamine that induces peripheral side effects but does not act on the central nervous system and thus does not affect the sleep EEG merits discussion. However, administration of an active placebo is problematical and must be debated for each study and for every substance to be tested.

Another general problem is the question of assigning patients to experimental groups. In many drug studies the assignment to groups is random. Frequently, however, practical limitations such as the number of patients available for the study, preclude random assignment. In these cases, a matching procedure has to be employed. In trials of hypnotic drugs groups must be comparable in age, sex, and length of previous illness, since, e.g., the duration of sleep and the delta sleep segment decreases physiologically with advancing age. Construction of different age groups (e.g., 20–35, 36–50, 51–65 years) within which each patient would be assigned at random to the experimental conditions is recommended.

Numerous hypnotic drug studies, especially long-term studies, must be conducted on an outpatient basis. Fundamentally, as stated earlier, polygraphic sleep registration is possible for this group. In this regard, it is necessary to control the compliance of the patients during the study. Qualitatively this can be achieved with the aid of medicament determination in urine or with the help of plasma level assays.

What are the specific problems that arise in designing a hypnotic drug study (Fig. 2)?

The ideal hypnotic drug would improve the quality of sleep, would cause no development of tolerance coupled with loss of efficacy, would possess no potential for addiction, would not trigger rebound insomnia upon discontinuation, would not cause impairment of daytime functioning, but would restore the disturbed sleep-wake regulation beyond the point of medicament intake. From these ideal

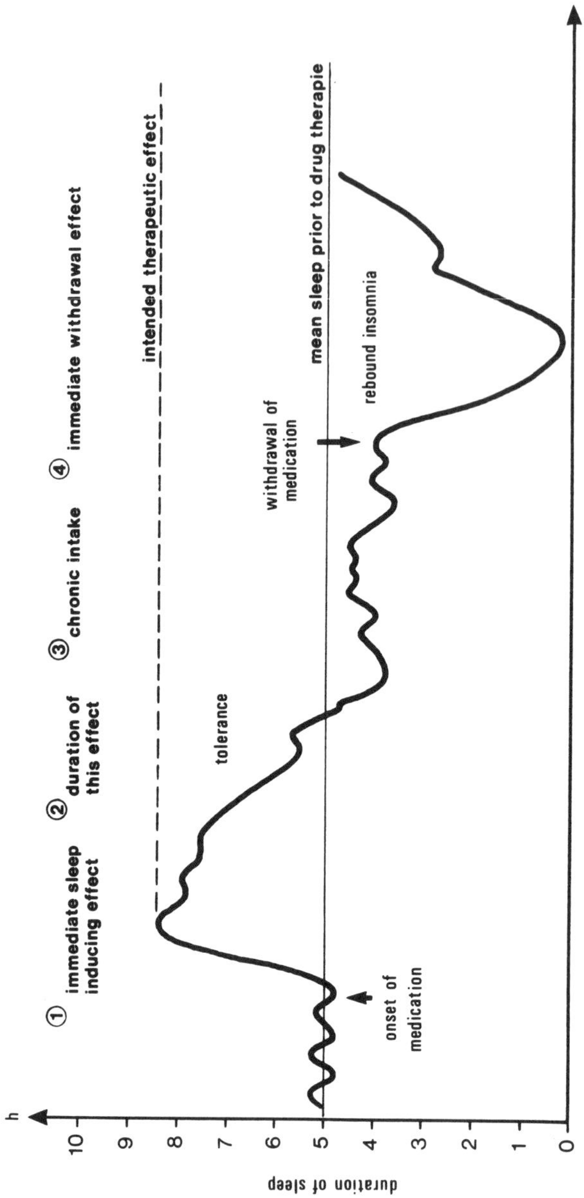


**Fig. 2.** Four questions to ask when evaluating hypnotic drugs (modified from Hauri (1982))

specifications (Hauri 1982) the following questions arise pertaining to the effects of the hypnotic drug:

1. Does the hypnotic drug induce sleep acutely in insomnia (Fig. 3a)?
2. Does a hypnotic drug take effect in chronic sleep disorders, i.e., does the hypnotic effect persist in the case of long-term intake or does tolerance develop and efficacy diminish (Fig. 3b)?
3. Does the effect of a hypnotic drug persist beyond the period of administration (Fig. 3e) or does the disturbed sleep-wake regulation return upon discontinuation (Fig. 3f) or does even rebound insomnia occur (Fig. 3g)?

The following study designs, which can be expanded or modified, are suited to providing answers to these questions.

The efficacy of a medicament can be tested most quickly and efficiently against placebo. The number of test persons necessary for a statistically significant

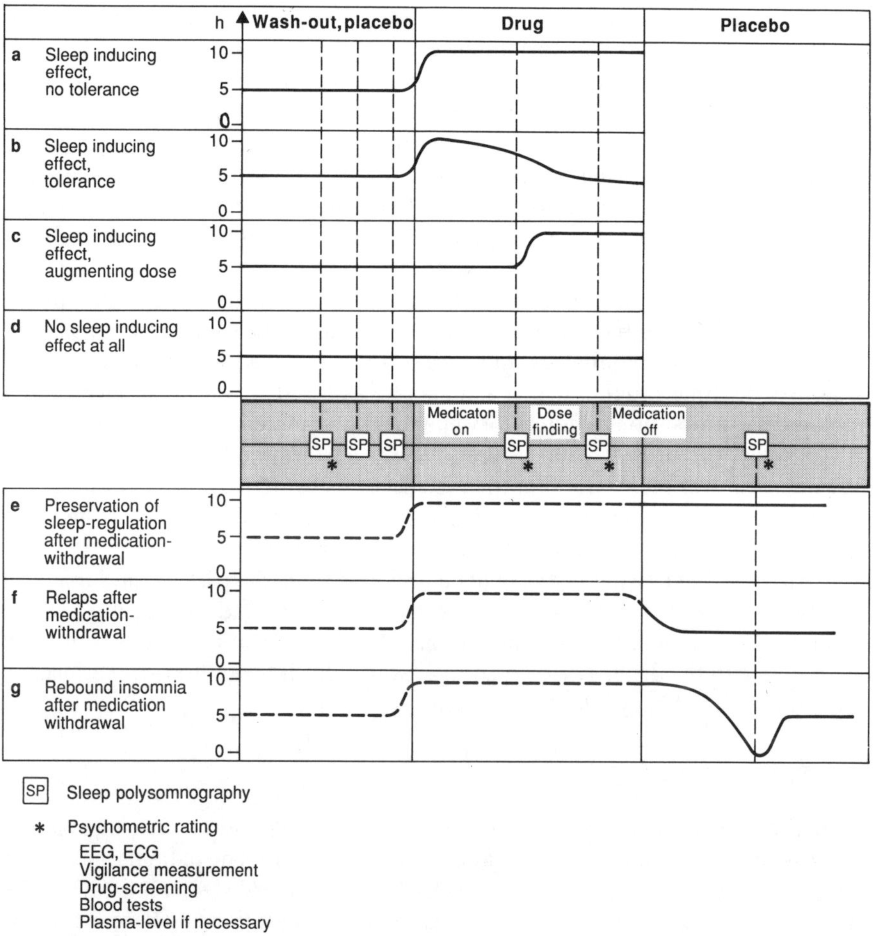


**Fig. 3a-g.** Study design specifications (see text)

statement is relatively low. For example, in order to show an improvement of 35% in the drug group vs the placebo group (with $\alpha$-error $\rho \leq 0.05$), each group must consist of only 16 patients. Beyond that, testing against placebo permits definitive differentiation between specifically clinical and pharmacologic effects of the test substance and nonspecific effects under placebo.

Two designs will be presented here.

## 6.1 The A-B-A Design

Patients must be drug-free at the beginning of the study. Frequently, the problem will be that only a stepwise reduction of the prior medication is feasible in order to prevent serious withdrawal complications such as cerebral seizures. If, for instance, benzodiazepines with half-lives of different length and different active metabolites are taken, a standardized procedure for the discontinuation process should be selected. Transforming the prior medication into the equivalent dosage of a benzodiazepine of medium-length efficacy without active metabolites is recommended (e.g., oxazepam). In the wash-out phase the medicament is slowly replaced by placebo until the patient is drug-free. Polygraphic sleep recordings during the initial hypnotic drug therapy and during the withdrawal phase provide data about the efficacy of the former therapy and the amount of rebound insomnia. An alternative is a slow, step-by-step reduction and discontinuation of prior medication before administration of placebo. After a wash-out phase of – if possible – at least 4 weeks the pharmacologically active substance is administered. Before the first sleep recording, urine analysis should prove that the patients are drug-free. After an adaptation night, two baseline nights in the sleep laboratory are recorded. In addition, the subjective judgment of sleep is quantified via questionnaires and visual analog scales; adjective mood lists quantify daytime fatigue, which can also be assessed by means of electrophysiological examinations. Laboratory chemical parameters are determined.

Finally, the drug is administered for a predetermined length of time. Following a control night, the therapeutic success is evaluated on the basis of the established criteria. In the case of an inadequate improvement of the sleep disorder, the dose is increased as discussed earlier (Fig. 3c).

After further treatment over a fixed period of time, sleep EEG and subjective ratings are repeated. Finally, the test substance is replaced by placebo and the sleep EEG examination after, for instance, 1 or 2 weeks of placebo is compared with that with the drug. The data comparison yields information on the specific, sleep-inducing effect of the test substance.

## 6.2 The A vs B Design

A further possibility involves testing the effect of an hypnotic drug in one patient group against the placebo effect in another patient group. The patients once again must be drug-free, if possible for 4 weeks. Prior to the first sleep registration, the above-mentioned parameters are established and adaptation and baseline nights are registered. Finally, patients are assigned to a drug or a placebo group and are treated over a defined period of time regularly for 3 or 4 weeks. During therapy, i.e., after approximately 4 weeks, a control night should be recorded to test the question of dose increase because of insufficient response. At the end of the study sleep EEG and subjective judgments of sleep quality are conducted. A comparison of drug data with those of the placebo group provides information on the efficacy of the hypnotic drug. Obviously, the value of this type of study increases if a placebo phase follows the drug phase to measure sleep quality after drug withdrawal.

In testing two active substances against each other, i.e., within the scope of a trial of a novel hypnotic drug against a standard medicament, substantially larger research groups of patients are necessary to arrive at statistically significant results because the differences between standard and test substances will be relatively slight in comparison with placebo. Moreover, special statistical procedures have to be chosen in order to control the type II error. Aside from the statistical problems arising with this type of study, there is also the problem of finding comparable doses in order to rule out the possibility that differences in efficacy and side effects are merely due to different doses. After an adequate wash-out phase both substances can be tested against each other in an A vs B design. Further difficulties arise when two pharmacologically different substances are tested against each other, such as, e.g., benzodiazepines versus antidepressants. Due to dissimilar characteristics such as development of tolerance, rebound insomnia, onset of efficacy, etc., problems of incomparability arise. A benzodiazepine may be more effective in immediate sleep induction, but may have disadvantages in regard to long-term application and withdrawal.

In view of the numerous methodological difficulties, comparative testing of two active substances against each other seems exceedingly problematical.

Regarding the long-term effect of hypnotic drugs, the study guidelines proposed up to now serve only to prove the acute pharmacogenic sleep inducing efficacy of a hypnotic drug and to quantify its intensity. A large number of difficulties relevant to the testing of hypnotic drugs and their long-term application are not covered by these guidelines. A major problem in therapy with hypnotic drugs is posed by the development of tolerance coupled with loss of efficacy, as in the prospective development of rebound insomnia following discontinuation of the medicament. These problems are especially important in the therapy of chronic cases of insomnia. To clarify the issue, examinations must be conducted over an extended period of time, say at least 1 to 2 months. To clarify whether chronic drug intake results in tolerance and loss of efficacy, corresponding collection of information, e.g., day time anxiety and performance, subjective well-being, nightmares, will be necessary in conjunction with sleep registration and a longitudinal design.

Regarding the quality of sleep after drug withdrawal, it is necessary to pursue the question of whether a hypnotic drug restores the disturbed sleep-waking regulation or whether rebound insomnia will develop upon discontinuation of medicaments. Thus, sleep must be registered under placebo upon completion of therapy. The sleep recording should take place after the drug has been excreted but in awareness of the length of its half-life. For most substances a polygraphic sleep recording can be made after approximately 14 days. A urine check will tell whether or not patients are drug-free.

In summarizing, a multitude of factors interfere with studies of hypnotic drugs and must be dealt with beforehand. The choice of the respective study design depends on the specific problem arising from the complexity of the phenomenon "sleep disorder." The aspects depicted here indicate the indispensability of certain requirements that must be met by hypnotic drug studies, but which have been neglected by many. They are vital to any conceptionalization of the intricacy of the problem.

## References

American Psychiatric Association (1987) Diagnostic and statistical manual of mental disorders. 3rd edn, Revised. APA, Washington DC

Association of Sleep Disorders Centers (1979) Diagnostic classification of sleep and arousal disorders. Sleep 2:1-137

Bixler O, Kales A, Soldatos CR, Kales J, Healey S (1979) Prevalence of sleep disorders in the Los Angeles metropolitan area. Am J Psychiatry 136:1257-1262

Bonnet MH, Webb WB, Barnard G (1979) Effect of flurazepam, pentobarbital and caffeine on arousal threshold. Sleep 1:271-279

Borbély AA (1986a) New techniques for the analysis of the human sleep-wake cycle. Brain Dev 8:482-488

Borbély AA (1986b) Benzodiazepinhypnotika: Wirkungen und Nachwirkungen von Einzeldosen. In: Hippius H, Engel RR, Laakmann G (eds) Benzodiazepine – Rückblicke und Ausblicke. Springer, Berlin Heidelberg New York, pp 96-100

Brownman CP, Cartwright RD (1980) The first-night effect on sleep and dreams. Biol Psychiatry 15:809-812

Buysse DJ, Reynolds CF III, Monk ThH, Berman SR, Kupfer DJ (1989) The Pittsburgh sleep quality index: a new instrument for psychiatric practice and research. Psychiatry Res 28:193-213

Carskadon M, Dement WC, Mittler MM, Guilleminault Ch, Zarcone VP, Spiegel R (1976) Self-reports versus sleep laboratory findings in 122 drug-free subjects with complaints of chronic insomnia. Am J Psychiatry 133:1382-1388

Chen CN (1979) Sleep, depression and antidepressants. Br J Psychiatry 135:385-402

Coates ThJ, George JM, Killen JD, Marchini E, Hamilton St, Thorensen CE (1981) First-night effects in good sleepers and sleep-maintenance insomniacs when recorded at home. Sleep 4:293-298

de la Pena A, Flickinger R, Mayfield D (1977) Reverse first-night effect in chronic poor sleepers. In: Chase MH, Mitler MM, Walters PL (eds) Sleep Research, vol 6. Brain Research Institute, UCLA, Los Angeles, p 167

EEC/CPMP Working Party on Efficacy of Drugs (1987) The conduct of clinical trials of medicinal products in the european community. III/411/87-EN Rev

Frankel BL, Coursey RD, Buchbinder R, Snyder F (1976) Recorded and reported sleep in chronic primary insomnia. Arch Gen Psychiatry 33:615-623

Guilleminault Ch (ed) (1982) Sleeping and waking disorders: indications and techniques. Menlo Park, California

Hauri P (1982) The sleep disorders, current concepts, scope, 2nd edn. Upjohn, Kalamazoo pp 31-32

Hofferberth B (1986) Saccadic eye movements as a measure of residual effects: temazempam compared with other hypnotics. Acta Psychiatr Scand [Suppl] 332:105-111

Ives JR, Woods JF (1975) 4-Channel 24 hour cassette recorder for long-term EEG monitoring of ambulatory patients. Electorencephalogr Clin Neurophysiol 39:88-92

Kales A, Soldatos CR, Bixler EO, Kales JD (1983) Rebound insomnia and rebound anxiety: a review. Pharmacology 26:121-137

Kamp A (1984) Long-term supervised domiciliary EEG monitoring in epileptic patients employing radio telemetry and telephone telemetry. II. Radio telemetry system. Electroencephalogr Clin Neurophysiol 57:584–586

Karacan I, Thornby JI, Auch AM (1976) Dose-related sleep disturbances induced by coffee and caffeine. Clin Pharmacol. Ther 20:682–689

Lohse MJ, Müller-Oerlinghausen B (1988) In: Schwabe U, Paffrath D (eds) Hypnotika und Sedativa. Arzneiverordungsreport 1988. Fischer, Stuttgart, pp 212–223

Lugaresi E, Zucconi M, Bixler E (1987) Epidemiology of sleep disorders. Psychiatr Ann 17:446–452

McGregor ED, Weitzman MD, Pollak MD (1985) Polysomnographic recording techniques used for the diagnoses of sleep disorders in a sleep disorder center. The Delta Recorder 21:1–13

Meyer-Ewert K, Wismans LL (1984) Vigilanzleistungen bei unbehandelten und behandelten Patienten mit Narkolepsie-Kataplexie. In: Kugler J, Leutner V (eds) Vigilanz-Ihre Bestimmung und Beeinflussung. Roche, Basel

Mittler MM, Gujavarty KS, Brownman CP (1982) Maintenance of wakefulness test: a polysonmographic technique for evaluating treatment efficacy in patients with excessive somnolence. Electroencephalogr Clin Neurophysiol 53:658–661

Ott H, Bischoff RC, Oswald I, Adam K, Fichte K, Heidrich H, Kubicki St, Stephan K (1985) Review of sleep induction and hangover effects with visual analogue scales. In: Kubicki St, Herrmann WE (eds) Methods of sleep research. Fischer, Stuttgart, pp 75–91

Rechtschaffen A, Kales A (eds) (1968) A manual of standardized terminology, techniques and scoring system for sleep stages of human subjects. Department of Health, Education and Welfare, Washington DC

Schmidt HS, Fortin LD (1982) Electronic pupillography in disorders of arousal. In: Guilleminault Ch (ed) Sleeping and waking disorders: indications and techniques. Menlo Park, California

Schramm E, Hohagen F, Graßhoff U, Berger M (1989) Strukturiertes klinisches Interview für Schlafstörungen nach DSM-III-R. Weinheim, Belz Verlag (in press)[2]

Soldatos CR, Kales JD, Scharf MB (1980) Cigarette smoking associated with sleep difficulty. Science 207:551–553

Spiegel R (1981) Sleep and sleeplessness in advanced age. In: Weitzman (ed) Advances in sleep research, vol 5. Spectrum, New York

Spitzer RL, Williams JB, Gibbons M (1986) The structured clinical interview for DSM-III-R. Biometric Research Department, New York State Psychiatric Institute, New York

Steiger A, Holsboer F, Benkert O (1987) Effects of brofaremine (CGP 11 305A), a short-acting, reversible, and selective inhibitor of MAO-A on sleep, nocturnal penile tumescence and nocturnal hormonal secretion in three healthy volunteers. Psychopharmacology (Berlin) 93:110–114

Trinder J (1988) Subjective insomnia without objective findings: a pseudo diagnostic classification? Psychol Bull 103:87–94

Tryer P (1988) Dependence as a limiting factor in the clinical use of minor tranquilizers. Pharmac Ther 36:173–188

van der Weide H, Kamp A (1984) Long-term supervised domiciliary EEG monitoring in epileptic patients employing radio telemetry and telephone telemetry I. Electroencephalogr Clin Neurophysiol 57:581–583

von Zerssen D (1986) Clinical self-rating scales (CSRS) of the Munich psychiatry information system (PSYCHIS München). In: Sartorius N, Ban T (eds) Assessment of Depression. Springer, Berlin Heidelberg New York

Webb WB, Campell SS (1979) First-night effect revisited with age as a variable. Waking and Sleeping 3:319–324

Westbrook Ph R, Keeman S (1986) Guidelines for multiple sleep latency test (MSLT): a standard measure of sleepiness. Sleep 9:519–524

Williams RL, Karacan I, Hursch CJ (1974) Electroencaphalography (EEG) of human sleep: clinical applications. Wiley, New York

Woods JH, Katz JL, Winger G (1987) Abuse liability of bezodiazepines. Pharmacol Rev 39:00

Yoss RE, Mayer NJ, Hollenhorst RW (1970) Pupil size and spontaneous pupilar waves associated with alertness. Drowsiness in sleep. J Neurol 20:545–554

---

[2] English version in prep.

# Placebo-Controlled Trials and Ethical Issues

# Placebo-Controlled Studies in Depression: Necessity and Feasibility

E.S. PAYKEL[1]

The general principles of drug evaluation in psychiatry have now been widely accepted, although it has taken some time for methodologies suitable for each specific situation to evolve and be refined, and further developments continue to occur. Comparison of a new antidepressant with a placebo is required before acceptance by most of the major national regulatory authorities, particularly the FDA, but is still questioned by some clinicians more than most aspects of trial design, so that it can be difficult to recruit sufficient investigators. The issues that it raises still therefore need separate consideration.

In this discussion I will focus particularly on antidepressants, although most of the issues also apply to other psychotropic drugs. I will first consider why placebo-controlled trials are needed, and will then examine ethical and practical issues.

## 1 Why Are Placebo-Controlled Trials Needed?

The possible scientific case against placebo-controlled studies is easily stated. Antidepressants have been available since the late 1950s. They are very effective and have transformed the treatment of depression. Their place and who responds to them are well known. Good methodology for their assessment in clinical trials is well established and universally accepted. It is neither ethically justified nor scientifically necessary to compare new drugs with a placebo: all that is needed is to show that they are as effective as standard drugs.

If this were all true, life would be much simpler for the antidepressant evaluator. Unfortunately, however, several of the statements on which it depends are at best questionable.

Before I consider the detail, I can best illustrate the case for placebo-controlled trials from two studies of my own, previously published. The first study measured change over time in two groups of depressives, treated with two different drugs in a randomised double-blind placebo-controlled trial (Paykel et al. 1968).The two drugs were imipramine and chlorpromazine. Both were given in a dose of 200 mg daily, for 3 weeks and they emerged showing no significant

[1] Professor of Psychiatry, University of Cambridge Clinical School, Addenbrooke's Hospital, Hills Road, Cambridge CB2 2QQ, United Kingdom

Methodology of the Evaluation of Psychotropic Drugs
Editors: O. Benkert, W. Maier, and K. Rickels
(Psychopharmacology Series 8)
© Springer-Verlag Berlin Heidelberg 1990

difference. The trial was the first one I conducted and was started 25 years ago, when the requirements for antidepressant studies were less well worked out. Sample sizes of 48 and 51 per treatment group were reasonably high but the patients, inpatients and day patients, tended to be rather chronic and resistant and the treatment period of 3 weeks was too short. The rating scales we devised for the study were not clearly validated, although they probably were adequate. There is other evidence that neuroleptics have some effect in depression (Overall et al. 1966) but, without a placebo group it is difficult to be convinced in retrospect that either drug was of much benefit in this study.

Figure 1 shows a second study. The two drugs seem comparable, with Drug B perhaps a little weaker than Drug A. Was either of benefit and did the difference, which was not significant in this rating, but did show up on one or two others, matter? Figure 2 provides the answer. This was in fact a three-group study, of amitriptyline (150–187.5 mg daily), phenelzine (60–75 mg daily) and placebo, given for 6 weeks, to outpatients with depression and mixed anxiety-depression (Paykel et al. 1982; Rowan et al. 1982). The striking finding was that both active drugs were superior to placebo and there was relatively little to distinguish them. The placebo group provided a marker that could not be dispensed with.

Why then is placebo comparison indispensable in evaluating efficacy of an antidepressant? First, the efficacy of antidepressants is limited. Figure 3 is a hypothetical diagram of the elements that might contribute to outcome in a patient or group of patients given an antidepressant drug.

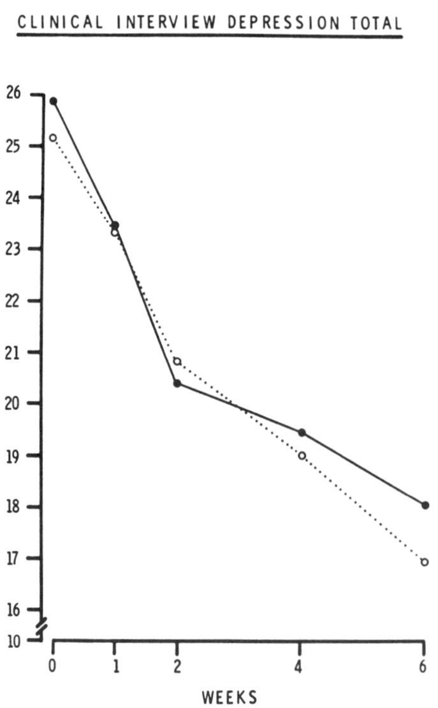


**Fig. 1.** Comparison of two drugs on a depression measure

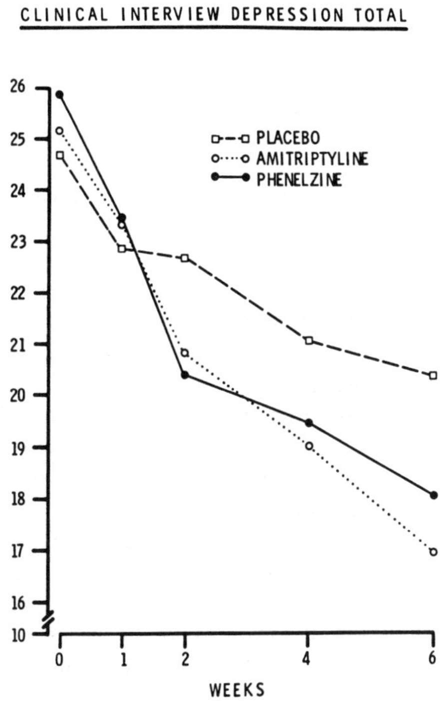


**Fig. 2.** The three drug groups from which Fig. 1 was derived

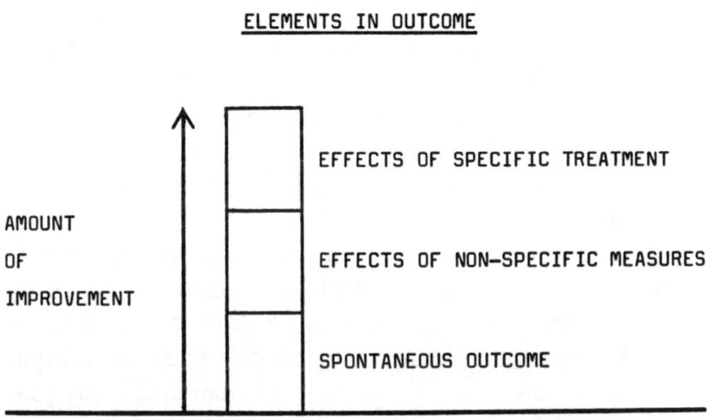


**Fig. 3.** Elements contributing to outcome on a specific treatment

First, recovery may have been spontaneous, reflecting the natural history of the disorder. We cannot now study spontaneous remission rates for the more severe forms of depression, since most reach treatment. However, history suggests that, long before modern treatments, depressions did improve: the remitting course of manic-depressive disorder was the basis of Kraepelin's separation of it from dementia praecox. Prevalence and episode rates for milder depression in the community, many of which are never recognised or treated, make it clear today that these remit.

Second, many other treatment processes are at work in a patient who receives an antidepressant, such as the perceived benefit of being able to ventilate one's problems to a sympathetic ear, the effect of coming into hospital with removal from stress and substitution of a supportive environment, the placebo effect of receiving even an inactive tablet. Actual placebo effects in depression are probably quite small (Paykel et al. 1975). However, the effects of other non-specific factors are probably quite strong, witness the considerable improvement which can occur in psychotic depressives during a drug-free week in a supportive ward environment.

Some quantification is available as to the effects of spontaneous remission and non-specific treatment factors combined. Morris and Beck (1974) reviewed evidence for the efficacy of the relatively small number of tricyclic antidepressants available in the USA in the early 1970s. There had been remarkably many placebo controlled trials – 93 in all. Among these, 61 had found drug superior to placebo, and 32 failed to. This gives good evidence for efficacy, assuming that all negative studies are published and studies use 5% significance. However, for one-third of studies to be negative is a substantial proportion. Part may be due to poor trial methodology, but part almost certainly reflects the modest therapeutic gains of the drugs. This is made clear by inspection of individual studies. In most trials, the proportion of the variance explained by active drug effects is modest. The proportion of recoveries on active drug in antidepressant trials is usually only about 30% higher than on placebo. This is exemplified, from our trial of phenelzine and amitriptyline (Rowan et al. 1982). The effects were mainly apparent in the proportions that improved a great deal; these comprised 18% on placebo, 43% amitriptyline, 41% phenelzine.

In circumstances where drug effects are modest, it will be easy for inclusion of inappropriate samples, inadequate doses, unsuitable rating scales, or inadequate treatment periods, to mask drug effects and prevent their demonstration. The appropriate samples are not easy to come by. Inpatients are increasingly selected by failure of prior drug treatment and likely to be resistant to further treatment. Increasing evidence indicates that severely psychotic and delusional depressives respond partly to antidepressants: better to ECT, or possibly, neuroleptics (Paykel 1988). On the other hand, mild depressives may show excellent recovery with spontaneous remission and non-specific treatment factors, leaving little room for drug-induced improvement.

Nor can good trial methodology be assumed. In particular, there is good evidence that 6 weeks is required to ensure demonstration of drug effects (Quitkin et al. 1984). Many studies still use shorter periods. The long treatment periods necessary and the general trend to improvement which is marked in most samples create further problems for drug-drug comparisons: short-term crossover studies are not possible.

Sample size is a crucial problem in many studies, if type 2 error is to be avoided. This is particularly so in drug vs drug comparisons where a new drug may have partial efficacy (Feinstein 1977; Altman 1980). In the usual parametric analyses of a continuous measure, critical ratios required for significance vary directly with magnitude of mean differences, but inversely with the square root of sample sizes. Thus, sample size required increases, in proportion to the square of the drop in the size of the expected difference, and very large samples are required for small differences.

The problem in doing without placebo comparison can be summarised simply: many factors mitigate against showing significant differences between treatments in depression. In a placebo comparison these factors act in a conservative direction: significance testing has to work against them. In a comparison between a new drug and standard antidepressant, the real hope is to find the new drug effective, and these factors aid in failure to find differences: type 2 error becomes crucial. The problem could be dealt with well if new drugs were only accepted if they were shown superior in efficacy to standard drugs, but no-one would take such a proposal seriously.

## 2 Other Psychotropic Drugs and Disorders

Space does not permit a full discussion of the issues in relation to other types of drugs and disorders, and these are dealt with fully in other papers in this volume. Briefly I would suggest that the same arguments apply with equal force in anxiety disorders: indeed the pendulum is swinging away generally from drug treatment of these disorders, at least in the UK. The main difference from depression is that short-term drug effects are easily demonstrable, so that more imaginative short-term crossover and latin square designs can be of value, rather than the parallel group designs necessary in depression.

In evaluating nootropics we do not yet have standard comparison drugs, and placebo expectancies, at least in relatives, can be high; so that the case for placebos hardly needs to be made. The biggest problems are perhaps in schizophrenia and mania. Here drug effects tend to be much larger and rapid in onset than in depression, spontaneous remission is much slower and response to nonspecific measures less marked, so that comparisons with placebo may be less essential. Level of disturbance may also be too great for ineffective treatment to be tolerable for long. Hirsch (elsewhere in this symposium) advocates placebo control in evaluation of new drugs in schizophrenia: the kind of short-term placebo control and placebo withdrawal study which he describes is equally applicable in mania.

## 3 Ethical Issues and Potential Disadvantages

Most arguments against use of placebo control groups concentrate not on the scientific but the ethical aspects. Although these are discussed by Helmchen (elsewhere in this volume), they require some consideration here, as well.

First, it should be noted that depression produces suffering for the individual, may produce harm to his or her work prospects, relationships, marriage and children, and may culminate in suicide. For the population as a whole this argues strongly in favour of the placebo-controlled study. Great harm can be done by widespread use of an ineffective substance claimed to be an antidepressant.

What of the subject in the study? Can it be justified to expose the individual to just these risks, for the sake of the group? I believe it is justified to do such studies, but with samples and under conditions where risk is minimised, in a way that does not apply in ordinary clinical use. I will deal more fully with the requirements to achieve this shortly. I would also emphasise that many patients with depression, extending well up into the moderate range of severity, are reluctant to take antidepressants and would like an opportunity to see if their depression will recover with other treatments but without an active drug. We find many patients in our own studies for whom the chance of not receiving active drug is a perceived advantage, facilitating recruitment into the study.

One must also consider other possible disadvantages in placebo-controlled studies. I do not think that there are many. Dropout rates may be higher than in drug-drug comparisons, since both subjects and staff are conditioned towards caution in the face of failure to improve: this may be an ethical benefit, but in fact the general trend to improvement in all groups, at least in outpatient antidepressant trials, is quite marked, so that dropouts due to treatment failure tend to be infrequent. In our own studies there have tended weakly to be higher dropout rates in active drug groups, due to side effects, rather than in the placebo group, due to treatment failure. Secondly, blindness may be harder to maintain, due to side effects on active drug. This is a real, but not usually a major problem; the incidence of "side effects" is surprisingly high in placebo groups, and sufficient to prevent confident guesses through the double blind.

Incorporation of a second comparison, with a known active drug, to make a three-group study, can be an advantage here, making it harder to spot the new drug. Its major advantage is an efficacy one: provision of a second marker group against which can be judged both efficacy of the drug, and behaviour of the trial itself in terms of efficacy demonstration, and I would strongly advocate such three-group designs as the standard.

## 4 Requirements for Placebo-Controlled Antidepressant Trials

For 20 years, since the late 1960s, I have been conducting antidepressant trials, almost all of them placebo controlled. I have set up for these purposes depression clinics successively in one centre in the USA and two in England. The studies have included trials of older antidepressants in acute (Rowan et al. 1982; Paykel et al.

1982) and maintenance treatment (Paykel et al. 1975) and in general practice (Paykel et al. 1988); studies of newer antidepressants in single centre studies (Norton et al. 1984) and in multicentre collaborations. My commitment to such studies, it will be evident, is strong, but equally strongly I believe in the importance of good and ethical patient care. A set of requirements enables the two to be combined in placebo-controlled studies. We are careful to specify these in detail in trial protocols, and have always found ethical committees, to whom all such studies are submitted, supportive and approving.

### 4.1 Full Informed Consent

Full informed consent is a sine qua non, as important to protect the researcher as it is vital for the subject. We use a written description of the study which the patient keeps, and written consent. Use of random assignment, of double blind conditions and of a placebo, are dealt with openly.

### 4.2 Careful Monitoring

Patients receive much more careful monitoring than is usual in routine practice, with detailed assessment and frequent contact. This is part of the implicit therapeutic contract in the research, which includes involvement of a team experienced in treating depression, close supervision and contact with a supportive therapeutic figure, and a commitment to continue treatment, with addition in due course after the study of whatever additional drugs and non-pharmacological, psychosocial and psychotherapeutic measures are necessary, to achieve recovery.

### 4.3 Right of Withdrawal

As important as the right of consent is the right of withdrawal, by patient or by investigator, at any point. This escape clause is vital, often rendering it easier to continue the individual patient in the study.

### 4.4 Selection of Appropriate Sample

An important element is selection of an appropriate sample. Subjects presenting major suicidal risk are automatically excluded. I have learned to be very cautious in including patients who have made recent suicidal threats or young patients under 25, who tend to overlap very much with overdosing suicide attempters in suicidal risk and tendency to drop out of treatment, and often show transient depression closely bound up with late adolescent relationships and behaviour problems for which a psychotherapeutic approach seems much more appropriate than a pharmacological one.

An important issue in sample selection concerns severity of depression. We tend not to include inpatients in placebo-controlled studies, although we do include them in drug-drug comparisons. Their distress is severe, rendering placebo administration less justified and harder to continue. They tend to be failures of earlier outpatient drug treatment, are more likely to be resistant to subsequent treatment. Other evidence increasingly indicates that psychotically and delusionally depressed patients respond poorly to antidepressants and better to ECT (Paykel 1988). On the other hand, the most mildly ill depressives may show too good an outcome without drugs. Leff (1973) suggested that the best subjects for treatment trials were intermediate in prognosis: poor prognosis patients tended to be too resistant to treatment, good prognosis patients not to need it.

Applying this to depression, outpatients of moderate severity make the best subjects, contrary to the view of some clinicians and regulatory bodies that the best subjects are hospitalised endogenous depressive inpatients. It is interesting that when Morris and Beck (1974), in their review of placebo-controlled tricyclic studies, broke down samples into outpatients and inpatients, it was outpatients who had the greater preponderance of positive studies (77%) as opposed to inpatients (62%). In a recent study of our own (Paykel et al. 1988) we examined the efficacy of amitriptyline against placebo in a relatively mild range of depressives, those treated in general practice in England. The threshold for superiority of drug over placebo extended surprisingly far into the mild range, to include patients with probable and definite major depression on the Research Diagnostic Criteria, but not minor depression, and to include all those with a score on the 17-item Hamilton Scale of 13 or more, but not those scoring 12 or less. Presence of endogenous features contributed nothing in this regard.

## 5 Conclusions

To conclude, placebo-controlled trials are an essential element in the establishment of efficacy of a new antidepressant. The magnitude of drug effects in depression is too small, variability in outcome too large, likelihood of either good remission due to natural course and non-specific treatment factors or of treatment resistant to drugs too high, risk of inadequate dose or treatment period too great, and of type 2 error generally too large, to depend safely on failure of demonstrating a significant difference from a standard drug. The simultaneous comparison with standard drug is a valuable adjunct. Placebo-controlled trials require care by the investigator, careful sample selection and monitoring, and a high standard of informed consent – but the whole field of drug evaluation is all the better for that.

## References

Altman DG (1980) Statistics and ethics in medical research. III. How large a sample? Br Med J 281:1336–1338

Feinstein AP (1977) Clinical biostatistics. Mosby, St Louis, chap 22

Leff JP (1973) Influence of selection of patients on results of clinical trials. Br Med J 4:156–158

Morris JB, Beck AT (1974) The efficacy of antidepressant drugs: a review of research (1958–1972). Arch Gen Psychiatry 30:667–674

Norton KRW, Sireling LL, Bhat AV, Rao B, Paykel ES (1984) A double-blind comparison of fluvoxamine, imipramine and placebo in depressed patients. J Affective Disord 7:297–308
Overall JE, Hollister LE, Johnson M, Pennington V (1966) Nosology of depression and differential response to drugs. JAMA 195:946–948
Paykel ES (1988) Antidepressants: their efficacy and place in therapy. J Psychopharmacol 2:105–118
Paykel ES, Price JS, Gillan RU, Palmai G, Chesser ES (1968) A comparative trial of imipramine and chlorpromazine in depressed patients. Br J Psychiatry 114:1281–1287
Paykel ES, DiMascio A, Haskell D, Prusoff BA (1975) Effects of maintenance amitryptyline and psychotherapy on symptoms of depression. Psychol Med 5:67–77
Paykel ES, Rowan PR, Parker RR, Bhat AV (1982) Response to phenelzine and amitriptyline in subtypes of neurotic depression. Arch Gen Psychiatry 39:1041–1049
Paykel ES, Hollyman JA, Freeling P, Sedgwick P (1988) Predictors of therapeutic benefit from amitriptyline in mild depression: a general practice placebo-controlled trial. J Affective Disord 14:83–95
Quitkin FM, Rabkin JG, Ross D, McGrath PJ (1984) Duration of antidepressant drug treatment. What constitutes an adequate trial? Arch Gen Psychiatry 41:238–245
Rowan PR, Paykel ES, Parker RR (1982) Phenelzine and amitriptyline: effects on symptoms of neurotic depression. Br J Psychiatry 140:475–483

# Ethical Problems and Design of Controlled Clinical Trials

H. HELMCHEN[1]

## 1 The Dimensional and Relational Character of the Problem

Psychiatry is rather far away from the therapeutic ideal (Ehrlich's *therapia magna sterilisans*): to achieve immediate and complete success in all patients with the disease for which the therapy is indicated (specific efficacy) with no undesired side effects (safety). Currently available psychiatric therapies achieve at best only moderate specific efficacy and safety, so therapy research in psychiatry is badly needed. The main tool for this is the controlled clinical trial. However, the vast number of trial types and designs indicates that there is no ideal for all questions, but only designs which are more or less appropriate for a specific question. Furthermore, a controlled clinical trial goes beyond the individual's therapeutic help insofar as it is an experimental procedure for gaining new knowledge and a more rational basis for improvement of therapy. According to the Helsinki/Tokyo Declaration this means a greater need for getting valid informed consent than in routine therapy. However, it is precisely from patients with psychiatric disorders that informed consent may be a particular problem. Although some psychiatric disorders may destroy the capacity of a patient to understand a given piece of information and to give valid consent, all psychiatrists know that this is, in contrast to common public opinion, by no means true of all psychiatric patients. Rather, in a considerable number of psychiatric patients the competency for full informed consent is reduced only transiently and/or partially, and in other patients full competency is maintained (Fletcher et al. 1985; Helmchen 1986a,b; Helmchen and Winau 1986).

From this we can conclude that none of the three main categories which are relevant in this context has a binary or black-and-white structure. Rather, these categories are dimensions, the validity of which in clinical trials can be established by a grading of the relationships between them:

- Trial: appropriateness of design
- Therapy: safety vs efficacy
- Informed consent: patients competence to understand complexity of trial, expected benefits of therapy, expected risks of therapy.

[1] Freie Universität Berlin, Psychiatrische Klinik und Poliklinik, Eschenallee 3, 1000 Berlin 19, FRG

Methodology of the Evaluation of Psychotropic Drugs
Editors: O. Benkert, W. Maier, and K. Rickels
(Psychopharmacology Series 8)
© Springer-Verlag Berlin Heidelberg 1990

Before going into more detail, let us note the following:

- The less the trial is to test hypotheses and the more it is to generate them,
- the higher the possible risks and the lower the expected efficacy,
- the more severe the psychopathological state and the lower the probability of full competence on the part of the patient, the more strictly the validity of informed consent must be checked.

## 2 Trial Design and Ethics

The first dimension is the trial. Its validity, and hence its results, depend on the appropriateness of its design for the question. This in turn depends on the type of question, e.g. whether the trial aims qualitatively at new therapeutic principles or mechanisms, or quantitatively at improvement of existing therapies, or, to put it into another perspective, whether the trial aims to generate or to test hypotheses. It also depends on the quality of the question, i.e. its accuracy.

For example, *duration of trial* depends on such considerations. If the trial is to test qualitatively whether a new therapeutic principle has any definable efficacy, e.g. cognitive efficacy of nootropics, then a longer trial duration, e.g. 12 weeks, may be necessary. If, however, the trial is to test quantitatively whether, for example, a new antidepressant drug will reduce the latency of onset of efficacy, then a duration of 2 weeks seems to be appropriate, because in that time the efficacy of existing standard therapies becomes apparent. A longer duration, e.g. more than 3 or 4 weeks in an antidepressant drug trial, may increase the drop-out rate and thus invalidate the results.

The accuracy of the question is most important for the calculation of the number of patients necessary for valid results. From an ethical point of view the investigator is obliged to formulate his questions as precisely as possible in order to avoid exposing more patients than necessary to the inconveniences and risks of a trial, such as side effects or lack of sufficient efficacy. Therefore the most recent guidelines for clinical drug trials, like the German *Grundsätze für die ordnungsgemäße Druchführung der klinischen Prüfung von Arzneimitteln* by the Federal Health Authority (BMJFFG 1987) call for biometrical justification of the sample size. Another way to keep the necessary *sample size* as small as possible is by valid trial strategies, e.g. sequential evaluation, which becomes more urgent the more likely severe the potential risks.

With regard to risks, *withdrawal criteria* have to be defined not only for the individual patient but also for the trial as a whole. This is because they may differ from each other and in the case of the trial include frequency as well as type and intensity of adverse events.

High *drop-out* rates not only burden these patients without achieving anything, but also at the very least extend the time needed to attain the designed sample size. They also have an impact on the representativity and also perhaps the comparability of the sample. Therefore, an upper limit for the number of drop-outs (e.g. 30%) should be defined and all influences arising from the design which may increase the drop-out rate should be minimized, e.g. by avoidance of both long wash-out and trial periods or of inappropriate selection criteria.

*Selection criteria* also provoke some cost-benefit considerations with regard to the validity of the trial, e.g. homogeneity of the trial population, in-patients or out-patients, severity of the psychopathological state or of the disease, and therapy-resistance (Angst et al. 1989). Criteria of homogeneity may not reflect sufficient homogeneity or be appropriate to the special investigational question. The first problem often seems to be relevant for psychopathological criteria, particularly if they can be seen as a final common pathway of different mechanisms. The second problem may be of significance in biological variables. These problems will be less significant in selection criteria for early phase clinical trials which aim to generate hypotheses, but will be more important for later phase trials which test specific hypotheses. However, to generate hypotheses from a less selected sample needs a larger sample size than for testing a specific hypothesis. This is in contrast to the established practice of clinical trials and therefore leads to results which, though significant, are not very specific. Furthermore, even in the case of selection criteria of sufficient homogeneity and appropriateness, the questions of generalizability, practical relevance and applicability of the results also have to be considered. It may be questioned, for example, whether it is appropriate to apply the results of clinical trials of antidepressant drugs in in-patients with severe states of depression to out-patients with mild depression.

From an ethical point of view, the criterion of *therapy-resistance* is of particular significance. In depression, for example, it is mainly used as an exclusion criterion. But this has to be challenged. Firstly, the problem of a generally accepted definition remains unsolved: should a depression be termed therapy-resistant with an unsuccessful therapy for 1 year or for at least 2 years; with one, two or more different antidepressant therapeutic principles; including or excluding ECT, psychotherapy, or combinations; and controlled or uncontrolled for adequate dose, drug plasma level, duration, and execution? Secondly, the need to overcome therapy-resistance, perhaps by new therapeutic principles, is much more urgent than to test a further antidepressant drug of an assumed known therapeutic mechanism for a questionable quantitative improvement of existing standard therapies.

It may be added that the exclusion of *spontaneous remitters* from clinical trials of specific therapies is well reasoned. But this must not lead us to exclude these patients from clinical therapy research. On the contrary, the neglect of research into autoprotective and self-healing mechanisms should be redressed.

Some of these considerations may add further aspects to the discussion of *placebo control* in antidepressant drug trials (Paykel, this volume). In Paykel's view out-patients are the most suitable depressive population for placebo comparisons. That way we can avoid the ethical problem of withholding an efficacious therapy from patients who need in-patient treatment due to severe depression, with vital or suicidal risks. Also, from the validity point of view, as mentioned above, this is desirable since the majority of depressives are treated on an out-patient basis. It is also necessary methodologically because of the high rate of spontaneous remissions and placebo reactions in out-patients. However, perhaps for that reason a clear placebo-verum difference in antidepressant drug trials in out-patients has not yet been established. On the other hand, this points to the possibility that accepted standard therapies of moderate and severe depression are no standards or are even ineffective in mild depression. The possible lack of an antidepressive standard therapy in out-patients with mild depression may be an additional argument for the ethical admissibility of the use of placebo in those patients. If some forms of antidepressive psychotherapy, e.g. cognitive or interpersonal forms, are to be accepted as standard therapy for such patients, then one has to deal with the methodological problems of testing drug therapy against psychotherapy, or of testing their combination. Practically, however, this seems advisable, because otherwise the majority of out-patients may not accept a placebo control. Our own experience shows that the participation of private practice psychiatrists in placebo-controlled trials is very low, and the drop-out rate of informed out-patients is very high. Information about patients on placebo control, however, is now generally accepted as an ethical need.

This problem probably could be overcome in patients with depressions resistant to standard therapies. Placebo control is acceptable in therapy-resistant depressions:

- Ethically because an efficacious therapy apparently does not exist
- Medically because sometimes withdrawal from all drugs is helpful
- Methodologically because spontaneous remission after longer duration of the depressive episode may be more probable.

Against these proposals, the prevailing concept of placebo-controlled antidepressant drug trials lies just in between, that is to take in-patients, for better compliance control, with moderate depressions (e.g. HDS $< 20$, $> 15$, without suicidality, anxiety etc.). If this is not acceptable for ethical reasons (withholding of efficacious therapy) and for methodological reasons (restricted representativity of such highly selected samples), and if the designs mentioned above cannot be followed for whatever reason, there remains no alternative but to test the experimental drug against a *standard drug*. However, in order to avoid both the beta-error and a large sample size, one must test for falsification of the zero hypothesis, i.e. that the experimental drug is an improvement with regard to either efficacy or to its quicker onset.

Against this strongly conservative position may be argued that the regulatory authorities in many EEC countries do not demand evidence of superiority of the experimental drug, only of its efficacy; nevertheless, the individual investigator can decide for himself to choose to define such criteria of superiority (e.g. more than 20% of efficacy, or significant improvement after 1 week). The (drug companies') argument that superiority cannot be defined only in terms of efficacy, but must also be defined in terms of safety or of the efficacy-safety ratio, is not valid in that to answer these questions other designs (mainly of phase IV) with much larger samples are necessary.

## 3 Therapy: Ethics of Safety Versus Efficacy

The second main dimension is therapy. The grading of its validity depends on the relation of safety to efficacy. An example is the trial proposed by Hirsch and Barnes (this volume) to test continuous low-dose neuroleptic versus intermittent neuroleptic maintenance therapy. From our own experience with such trials, it seems clear that the relapse prophylactic efficacy of intermittent therapy is less than that of continuous treatment, as well as that safety is higher in the former, the influence of which on well-being, social behaviour, and compliance is still being studied. Grading of efficacy, according to frequency, intensity, and quality of relapses, and of safety, also by frequency, intensity, and type of side effects, may serve as a basis for a quasi-quantitative estimation of the safety-efficacy ratio, the grade of which can be used as a definition of the validity of the therapy. From an ethical point of view such a design has to be justified (and documented) comprehensively and explicitly by the investigator, not only for his own benefit but also for the information of the patient.

## 4 Informed Consent

The third main dimension is informed consent. The grading of its validity depends on the relationship between several variables. This is exemplified by Alzheimer's dementia. No efficacious therapy is available for this condition, but it is particularly badly needed (Helmchen et al. 1989). However, therapy research in the majority of such cases is not admissible, because at least in more progressed stages of Alzheimer's dementia the capacity of informed consent is destroyed. Nevertheless, this capacity too has by no means a yes or no structure; rather, it is a dimension which can be graded. The grading is based on an estimation of the capacity to understand and to process information, and to decide and to behave more or less reasonably. The grading procedure itself can be viewed also as dimensional, and it may be added that these grades are, of course, dependent on stage and severity of the dementive process.

Grading of capacity for informed consent:
- Full capacity
- In spite of the (status) diagnosis, no (functional) restriction of capacity exists
- Capacity is preserved for simple decisions
- Capacity is abolished legally but preserved actually and with regard to a factual decision (assent)
- Capacity is abolished legally and actually.

The grading of the capacity for informed consent is related to complexity of information and significance, as well as probability of both expected efficacy and risks. All these variables themselves can be subjected to a grading. Thus, for example, the grading of side effects mentioned above can be seen as only a section of a dimensional scale of risk. According to the criteria of risk estimation (defined by the individual's physical and psychic integrity, civil rights, and dignity), its endpoints can be defined as unacceptable risks, in extreme cases death, irreversible damage, and severe pain, and risks or inconveniences generally accepted as minimal, such as those which are inherent to routine investigations or daily life activities. Finally, some prerequisites of risk estimation are common sense, experience on the part of the investigator, statistical epidemiological data, and full knowledge of the subject's circumstances.

## 5 Conclusion

From an ethical point of view the conclusion is that the investigator should know about the special ethical problems of his design, the involved and conflicting values of human value systems in, for example, placebo control in the case of an existing standard therapy for a severe disorder such as depression. But first and foremost, the clinical trial investigator has to have sound scientific and professional standard. He has to be qualified to do the following:

- Check that the trial design is appropriate
- Explain in detail the anticipated risks and benefits
- Evaluate adequately the validity of informed consent.

These abilities and knowledge, plus the investigator's adequate experience of routine therapy, are necessary for designing and executing the controlled clinical trial in an appropriate ethical manner.

This means that a controlled clinical trial is justified only if the design is qualified to give a clear-cut answer. Therefore it seems ethically doubtful to use trial designs the appropriateness of which the investigator, due to incompetence or neglect, has not checked himself.

## References

Angst J, Hippius H, Woggon B et al. (1989) Consensus conference on the methodology of clinical trials in antidepressants. Pharmacopsychiatry 22:3–7

BMJFFG (Der Bundesminister für Jugend, Familie, Frauen und Gesundheit) (1987) Bekanntmachung von Grundsätzen für die ordnungsgemäße Durchführung der Klinischen Prüfung von Arzneimitteln. Bundesanzeiger no 243, p 16617, 30 Dez 1987

Fletcher JC, Dommel FW Jr, Cowell DD (1985) Consent to research with impaired human subjects. IRB: A Review of Human Subjects Research 7 (6):1–6

Helmchen H (1986a) Aufklärung, Einwilligung. In: Müller C (ed) Lexikon der Psychiatrie, 2nd edn. Springer, Berlin Heidelberg New York, pp 79–80, 221–222

Helmchen H (1986b) Ethische Fragen in der Psychiatrie. In: Kisker KP, Lauter H, Meyer J-E, Müller C, Strömgren E (eds) Psychiatrie der Gegenwart, vol 2: Krisenintervention, Suizid, Konsiliarpsychiatrie. Springer, Berlin Heidelberg New York, pp 310–368

Helmchen H, Winau R (eds) (1986) Versuche mit Menschen. De Gruyter, Berlin, p 391

Helmchen H, Kanowski S, Koch HG (1989) Forschung mit dementen Kranken: Forschungsbedarf und das Problem der Einwilligung. Eth Med 1:83–98

# Biostatistics and Measurement of Drug Effects

# Statistical Issues: Sample Size and Dropout

P. Lavori[1]

## 1 Introduction and Plan of the Chapter

Psychopharmacology has reached a state of maturity characterized by the availability of "standard" treatments of proven efficacy (relative to placebo), for many of the most common mental disorders. That has caused an evolutionary saltus in the kinds of research designs contemplated for studying the efficacy of compounds. Because of the need to compare the new treatment with the standard, studies with at least two "active" treatment conditions have become more frequent. For reasons that will be discussed below, many researchers find it desirable (or even necessary) to retain the placebo condition in the design, and place great weight on the results of the contrast between placebo and standard. Thus, the first jump in the evolution of clinical trials design has usually been the "three cell" design (two actives and a placebo cell).

Given the role of the placebo-standard contrast as a "calibrator" of the validity of the study, the consequences of a type 2 error (failing to detect a true difference as statistically significant because of sampling variation) are severe. Thus, it may be thought wise to plan a large enough sample size that this error rate is held to 10% or lower, rather than the more customary 20%. The consequences of this are discussed below.

The comparison between the two active conditions (standard and innovation) may be expected to have a small true size (i.e., the expected difference between the active treatment groups may be much less than the expected difference between either one of them and the placebo group). This also has an effect on the necessary sample size, as discussed further in this chapter.

Many researchers find the placebo cell increasingly problematic, especially in the depressive and anxiety disorders, precisely because of the expectations aroused in patients and clinicians by the availability of well-tested "standard" treatments. The often surprising "efficacy" of placebo in controlled trials helps to keep this option alive, but also poses a dilemma for the researcher, since many researchers believe that placebo effects of varying sizes may not simply add to treatment effects, leading to distortions in estimates of treatment effects. This is taken up in detail below.

[1] Massachusetts General Hospital, Harvard Medical School, Cambridge, MA, USA

**Methodology of the Evaluation of Psychotropic Drugs**
Editors: O. Benkert, W. Maier, and K. Rickels
(Psychopharmacology Series 8)
© Springer-Verlag Berlin Heidelberg 1990

Testing adjuvant therapies, or changes in the conditions of therapies, are also areas of increasing interest. These "two factor" problems lead to considerations of interaction, a concept that has a precise meaning in statistics that is discussed below. Multifactor experiments have extra benefits and complexities that are also taken up below. The issue of placebo nonadditivity is seen to be a special case of the factorial problem, sometimes hidden in multisite trials in the site main effect and interactions with treatment. These concepts are also related to the discovery of "indications" for treatment (subgroups of patients for whom the different treatment recommendations are made). The potential savings offered by factorial designs in a coordinated strategy of investigation are discussed.

Trends toward larger and more complex trials make the issue of nonsampling errors more salient than ever. This is discussed in Sect. 11, and one potential source of important bias, dropout or nonadherence, is discussed. The goals and properties of several strategies for estimation of treatment effects (in the presence of dropout) are explored, and references are provided to recent statistical work on the "missing data" problem.

## 2 Recent Trends in Design of Clinical Trials in Psychopharmacology

In the United States, industry-sponsored clinical trials of "innovations" (i.e., proprietary compounds) predominate in phase 3 trials in psychopharmacology, involving the greatest number of trials with the largest samples of patients and the most money. Although other funded research (mostly NIMH-supported) has an influence out of proportion to the resources devoted to it, until (or unless) the research priorities in this area change, the modal clinical trial will involve an industry sponsor and an "innovation" (perhaps a new use for an old drug). It will take place in a complex environment of regulation and publication defined by the double audience of the Food and Drug Administration scientist-regulators and the investigators' peers in the academic and medical community who comprise the reviewers, editors, and readers of medical journals. The peculiar strains imposed by this "double life" include a very strong incentive to satisfy the desire of regulators and many of their peers in clinical research to see the results of an internal placebo-controlled test of the efficacy of a standard treatment as well as a contrast of the innovation with the standard. The often-repeated basis for this requirement for a placebo cell is that a failure to find a placebo-standard difference casts doubt on the validity of the experiment and makes it impossible to interpret a null finding between the active conditions. The argument reflects the idea that an apparent finding of "equivalent efficacy" may be impossible to distinguish from poor experimental technique unless the study has such a successful built-in calibrator. The sponsor of a clinical trial may hope for rough equivalence in efficacy between the (proprietary) innovation and the standard treatment, with some advantage in tolerance or other ancillary benefit in favor of the innovation. Under the present circumstances of regulation, as expressed by Dr. Paul Leber of the FDA (1988 NCDEU conference, Key Biscayne), the sponsor will meet a very cold reception unless the study provides the expected (statistically significant) advantage of standard treatment against an internal placebo group, as well as a significant innovation advantage over placebo. Effectively, the two-group active-active trial is limited to the (rare) case that the sponsor expects the innovation to (significantly) beat the standard.

## 3 How Much Power?

This state of affairs may make it necessary to consider setting type 2 error rates lower than the customary 20% in the calculation of sample size requirements. First, since the consequences of a type 2 error in the placebo-standard contrast are so catastrophic, it may be thought wise to set that parameter to 10% or lower (i.e., determine sample size using a design power of 90% for the placebo-standard contrast). Second, there are now two contrasts with placebo to worry about, and the opportunity for chance variations in sample compositions is increased, with attendant increase in the risk of a false overall "null" result. That is, by chance one may miss the expected standard-placebo difference, and therefore have an uninterpretable study, or this contrast may succeed and the innovation-placebo contrast may fail by chance. A study that is designed with 80% power for each of the contrasts separately will actually have a somewhat lower power to detect the composite alternative that standard and innovation have the same positive advantage over placebo. By a (conservative) calculation that ignores the cor-

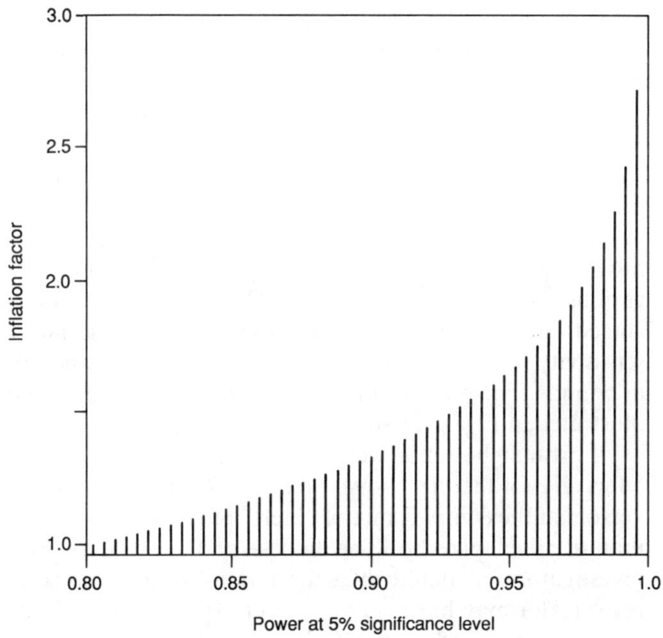


**Fig. 1.** Inflation of sample size as power is increased

relation of the two contrasts, it can be seen that changing the design power to 90% will provide at least 80% power overall.

At a given type 1 error rate and population distributional parameters, the effect of a change from 20% to 10% type 2 error is to multiply the required sample size (per group). The "inflation factor" (by which the sample must be multiplied) for the alpha level of 5%, as the power (100%-type 2 error rate) is raised from 80% toward 100%, is expressed in Fig. 1, which is based on the normal-theory calculation presented by Fleiss (1986). Furthermore, the desire to hold experiment-wise type 1 error rates down (the multiple comparisons problem) may lead investigators to increase the critical ratio (for the $t$ statistics of the contrasts), thus requiring a further inflation of the sample size to reduce the nominal type 1 error rate. A more general reason for designing to a lower type 1 error rate (alpha) for the active-active contrast stems from the fact that the standard treatment is subject to a repeated contest with each new innovation, and it would be highly undesirable to have a false positive result appear in any of these contrasts. From a social point of view, the "hard-won" status of "standard" should not be lightly discarded or jeopardized.

## 4 How Large is the Effect?

Designers of experiments often describe relative differences between treatments by the difference in some outcome measure (a score or rate) divided by the standard deviation of that measure. (In design of experiments, the standard deviation is often assumed, sometimes optimistically, to be the same for all treatment conditions, while in other areas, such as meta-analysis, the standard deviation of the "control" condition is taken as the denominator, in which case the ratio is called an effect size). The observed value of a test statistic (such as Student's $t$, which is the observed difference divided by the estimated standard error of that difference) in an experiment will usually be tested for "significance", usually at some conventional level (5% or 1%), by comparing it to a "critical value." For any rate of type 2 error (failing to detect a true difference, false null result), the statistician may calculate a sample size necessary to detect various values of that ratio (d). The power calculation thus involves a balanced decision among lowering the risk of a false null result, increasing the sensitivity of the experiment to lower levels of (d), and keeping the sample size in bounds. The relationship of the sample size to the standardized difference is illustrated in Fig. 2 for 90% power at 5% alpha.

Fortunately, one is likely to have reasonably good estimates of the population effect size for the placebo-standard contrast, at least for some sort of "average" version of the complex mix of "inert" pill and background clinical management that is called placebo. The hopes (and previous work) of the sponsor and investigators will define the expectations for the innovation-placebo effect. The investigator may have very different expectations for the active-active comparison, and this is reflected in different conclusions about the required sample sizes in the active and placebo cells.

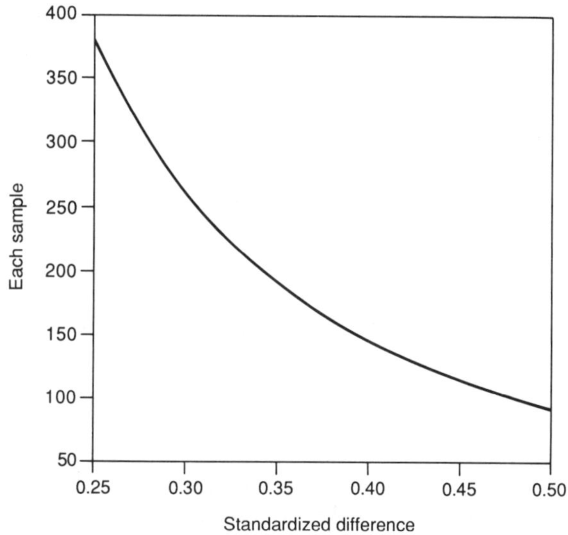


**Fig. 2.** Relationship of sample size to the standardized difference

Effect sizes among active treatments may be small. The innovation may differ from the standard in a subtle way, such as a small change in formulation intended to reduce a side effect, or a chemical alteration of the basic compound that has some promise for a wider spectrum of activity. Since psychiatry does not yet have the means to predict who will be "resistant" to a standard treatment, it is difficult to design trials in which to test the possibility of wider activity, by analogy to the tests of alternatives to penicillin in Gram-negative infections. Thus, any innovation has a steep hill to climb. It usually must "compete" with the standard on its "home ground." The standard may be familiar to patients and clinicians, and may have good acceptance. The innovators may not yet have a good "target group" of illnesses in which to test the innovation. All of these considerations lead to the likelihood that there will be small effect sizes in trials that test innovations against standard, unless the standard is very weak or the innovation is a true "breakthrough." But psychopharmacology is a mature field, with strong standard treatments for many illnesses, and a corresponding absence of recent breakthroughs. In a mature therapeutic area, emphasis shifts to modest "engineering" improvements rather than major breakthroughs. Investigators may hope for equivalent efficacy with improved safety or acceptability of the innovation. Gilbert et al. (1977) have reported that most innovations in medicine and surgery have very modest expectations against "standard," and they interpret this as a consequence of the state of development of these fields of medicine. This is also characteristic of psychopharmacology today. The investigator and sponsor ought to be very sure in advance whether their goal is to demonstrate that the innovation is "very nearly as good as" standard (i.e., the advantage of standard is unlikely to be greater than some small preset figure-of-merit), or (more ambitiously) that the experiment must have high power to detect an expected small advantage of the innovation. An example of the former case is the NIMH collaborative lithium study (Gelenberg et al. 1989), in which the intent was to set narrow confidence bounds around what was expected to be a small observed difference in relapse rates between low and standard dose conditions. This expectation leads to a consideration of the problem in terms of widths of confidence intervals, and to related issues in "equivalence" testing. The second case extends the more usual power/significance testing approach into the domain of small effects. The sample size requirements are strongly affected by this change in focus, from large to small effects, since the sample size is generally proportional to the square of the reciprocal of the effect. Thus, halving the effect size quadruples the sample, as can be seen in Fig. 2.

Thus, the clinical experimental comparison of active treatments (especially if one of them is a standard treatment), will almost surely involve smaller effect sizes, and therefore larger samples, than otherwise similar trials of active versus placebo. When the two are merged, as in the three-group experiment comparing innovation, standard, and placebo, the computation of required sample size becomes entangled in the issues of different effect sizes. It may be necessary in some experiments to consider the power requirements for the various contrasts separately. Much work of a technical statistical nature has been done on this problem; it will be a major challenge to use this work to inform future planning of experiments in psychopharmacology.

## 5 An Ethical Dilemma

It is implicit in the above discussion that it is in the investigator's (and sponsor's) economic interest to create a context that favors as large an expected active-placebo contrast (effect size) as possible, since small effect sizes will lead to large samples. However, a large (expected) effect size carries an ethical burden, since the investigator now strongly believes the placebo patients will be at a disadvantage, relative to the standard group. In order to minimize this difference, the investigator may work with a more "active" form of placebo, (as discussed below), and thus incur costs by requiring larger samples. Patients, and their advocates, will quite reasonably expect the investigator to bear some of the burden of experimentation, to the extent that there are choices to be made among different versions of the placebo condition.

## 6 How Active is Your Placebo?

As has been so eloquently argued by Parloff (1986), the notion of a singular, inert, devitalized "placebo" in psychiatric research is nonsense.

"If the problem requiring treatment is primarily a disorder of cognition, mood, behavior, or personality, then it is difficult to conceive of any nonspecific therapist-patient interaction as inert. If the disorder may be characterized as nonspecific in its nature and perhaps in its etiology – that is, perception and interpretation of unfortunate and noxious social relationships – then perhaps effective treatment can also be nonspecific, involving amelioration by favorable relationships with the therapist" (Parloff 1986).

The simple "sugar pill" is augmented by many "nonspecific" effects (some of which have names). Such effects may arise from the intense study of patients in trials (a kind of incidental, unofficial psychotherapy) or from extraordinary efforts made to induce patients to enter or remain in placebo-controlled studies. At the least, a truly inert placebo condition may jeopardize recruitment and retention, since it may involve perceived sacrifices (such as giving up psychotherapy, behavior therapy, occasional medications, or other valued treatments forbidden by the study protocol). It might also involve reducing systematically the opportunities for rapport and empathy between patient and clinician, which would certainly be expected to affect retention in studies. But why should the investigator believe that a "strong" placebo will lead to a small effect (active-placebo contrast)? Why would the active groups not be lifted by the same tide?

## 7 Patient-Defined Placebo

Some of the ethically desirable features of a "strong" placebo condition may come from a flexibility of choice offered to the patient. If patients do not have to give up their therapists or their "prn" beta-blockers or anxiolytics, they will be happier, and they may have better outcome as well. However, if patients who are not satisfied with the results of their therapy are more likely to use these options, and if these options are actually helpful, then such patient-chosen (variable) placebo conditions will cause an underestimate of any true effect of treatment. The extreme case of this option is that the patients may take the standard medication if they are not satisfied with their assigned treatment. Of course, the investigator may restrict the protocol, and "trade" with the patient by offering a very attractive fixed background of clinical management. Why should this cause a shrinkage of effect size?

## 8 Is There a Ceiling to the Benefit?

If the patients make use of the background clinical management to a degree that depends on how well they perceive themselves to be doing, then the placebo condition is not really fixed, and the problem discussed in the preceding paragraph remains. With great effort, the investigator may succeed in minimizing this variation, perhaps by vigorously pursuing the background therapy in a very structured way. Many investigators believe that the problem with strong placebo would still remain. This is sometimes expressed as a "ceiling on benefit"; either there is only "so far to go" in an individual patient, so that once the placebo achieves that level there is no further advantage to be found, or (more likely) there

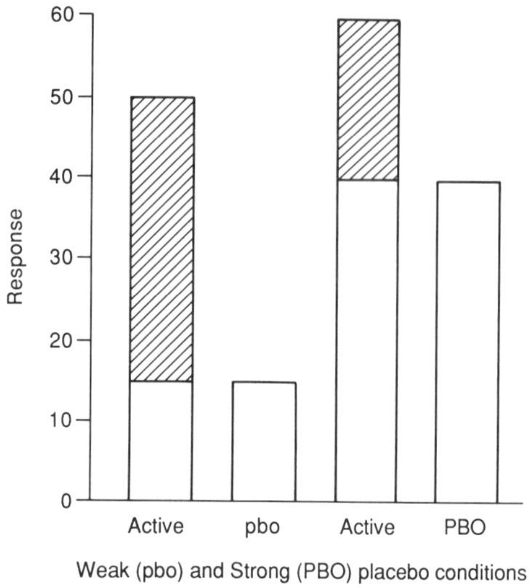


**Fig. 3.** Effects of placebo and active treatment

are only a fixed proportion of "curable" cases, and as the placebo condition captures more and more of them, there is less "head-room" for the active condition. In this view, to the extent that placebo effects are large, treatment differences may be distorted, since these effects and the active effects may not simply add (Fig. 3). Failure of additivity implies that the treatment effect would be estimated differently in a trial with a different placebo condition, complicating interpretation. This dilemma creates a difficult ethical situation, as it pits the investigator's interests (weak placebo) against the patient's (good expectation of success).

It should be emphasized that there is not much empirical evidence for or against this position. Perhaps a reasonable recommendation is that investigators should bring some research to bear on the effect of placebo strength on estimation of treatment efficacy. The methodology for such research turns out to involve the concept of factorial design, which is taken up next.

## 9 Treatments and Factors

The fundamental question raised above is whether changes in the level of background clinical management affect the observed consequence of adding a particular "active" treatment condition. For example, one may have two levels of contact with study personnel: occasional and intensive, and patients might be randomized to these levels and also randomized to pill-placebo or active compound. The main paradigm for studying the combination of several factors (in the example these are the active vs pill-placebo factor and the factor defined by level of contact) is the factorial design, with analysis of variance as the main tool for statistical analysis. The question raised above can then be rephrased statistically as an inquiry into the existence of a "statistical interaction" between the treatment and the "contact factor." Contrary to common usage, this term has a specific meaning in experimental design. At each level of the "contact" factor, one obtains an estimate of the effect of the drug treatment (by subtracting the means, for example). Thus, the "effect" of treatment at low contact level is the difference in average response between the low contact, active drug group and the low contact, pill-placebo group, while the "effect" of treatment at high contact is the difference in average response between the high contact, active drug group and the high contact, pill-placebo group. The difference in these two "effects" is the statistical interaction. The reader will verify by algebra that the statistical interaction is identical when the roles of the "treatment" and the "contact factor" are reversed in the above calculation. This interaction can be tested for statistical significance against the null hypothesis that the interaction is zero by standard methods (Fleiss 1986).

The interaction is sometimes called synergy or potentiation of one treatment by another (or by a factor) when the joint effect is greater than the sum of the individual effects, and it is this possibility that holds the greatest interest for the investigator. It seems, however, that the reverse possibility is more common. For example, when a clinical trial of drugs is proposed, there is seldom much consideration given to the possibility of defining the base treatment level as including psychotherapy (although "forbidding" therapy may make the study harder to do). The common view is that increasing the base level of therapy may decrease the size of the active-placebo or active-active effect. This implies a negative interaction between the base level of therapy (clinical management) and the other treatment factors. This may well be the case; one implication is that the idea of the treatment effect becomes multivalued, since the treatment effect size is thought to be influenced by the background value of the clinical management provided to the patients. This background level of treatment surely varies among trials; more likely it varies within trials (between sites, physicians, etc.) as well. If the level of "placebo" interacts with the treatment being studied, this is an important thing to measure, as the effect of treatment will depend on the context in which it is applied. Rather than a nuisance, the "problem" of varying strength of placebo is a key part of the entire picture of efficacy. In this view, the placebo strength problem is a special case of the more general issue of testing combinations of treatments.

Another hallmark of the maturity of the field is the increased interest in testing combinations of treatments, including primary and adjuvants, mixed mode therapies (behavioral and pharmacologic treatments, for example), and variations in ancillary conditions (e.g., duration of treatments). There are two main reasons for using multiway designs for studying combinations of treatments. First, the investigator may be interested in the interaction of two treatments on outcome. If one seeks to measure interactions, a factorial design is indicated; one cannot measure interactions without multifactor trials. Indeed, in order to combine estimates of individual treatment effects from separate single-factor trials into an estimate of the joint effect of the treatments one must assume additivity (lack of interaction). That leads to the second reason for considering factorial designs. In the absence of interaction among the factors, great increases in efficiency of estimation can be purchased at a discount in sample size. It is possible to estimate the effects of several factors in a single factorial trial with much less than the total number of patients required in individual trials of each factor. This is more than an "economy of size," since the advantage scales with the dimension of the design.

Thus, the proliferation of several individual single factor designs is an inefficient (and possibly misleading) strategy for understanding joint effects of treatments. It relies on an assumption for correctness that can only be tested in a factorial design, and if the assumption is correct then it is less efficient than a factorial design. The only justification for the series of single-factor trials is simplicity, but that simplicity also means limited reach.

## 10 Who Should Receive What Treatment?

The discovery and determination of "indications" depends on the analysis of interactions; to determine that patients with panic and depression should receive drug X while patients with panic alone should receive drug Y one must show the existence of a particular kind of interaction between the treatment level (X or Y) and the patient factor "comorbid depression." This kind of analysis is formally similar to the analysis of factorial experiments, although the interpretations of the "effects" of "factors" such as sex, age, subtype, or comorbidity will be different from the interpretation of the effect of a treatment.

Thus, researchers in psychopharmacology will need to consider new strategies for design and analysis of clinical trials of efficacy that respond to the alternatives embodied in comparisons of active treatments actively competing with each other. This stage of development involves a corresponding shift toward more complex and subtle differences in efficacy. It also raises the costs and difficulties by manyfold, with consequently greater risks and costs of failure and error. This seems to be the inevitable concomitant of progress.

## 11 Bias Versus Variance

As sample sizes grow and designs become more expensive, study results become more precise and influential, raising the possibility of a very precise and convincing answer that is grossly incorrect. In statistical terms, the overall performance of an estimate of an effect is determined by two components: the accuracy of the estimate (if I did the experiment over and over would the average estimate approximate the true effect?) and the precision of the estimate (how much can an individual trial result be expected to vary from the long-run average of such results?). Precisely, the expected squared error is the sum of the variance (sampling error) of the estimate, and the square of the bias. The sampling variance is reduced proportionately to the sample size, while the bias does not change, so that in large studies the bias (systematic error) grows in relative importance.

Bias reduction comes from good technique, including randomization, masked assessments, careful planning of analysis, and interpretation of results relative to the appropriate population. For example, differential dropout may bias comparisons of treatments, and this problem just gets worse as the sample size increases. Thus, the usual practice of "padding" the sample (or adaptively recruiting) is inadequate at best, and may increase bias at worst.

I will concentrate my discussion here on the choice of analysis in the presence of moderate differential dropout, since I think that this is a relatively unexplored part of the problem described above, which is in some ways peculiar to psychopharmacology research. I assume the following context:

1. Dropout rates are large enough to matter but not so large or variable that they completely preclude further analysis. If the dropout rates in two treatment groups are only 3% vs 5%, and the difference in an outcome such as "recovery" is 60% vs 40% (as measured, say, in adherors), there is no issue, since no important effects could be concealed by such low and similar rates of dropout. If instead the dropout rates in the groups are 70% and 10% then the conclusion may be determined completely by the decision about what to do with the dropouts.
2. No post-drop measurements are available in patients who did not complete the protocol. Thus, dropout is a censoring variable. If all outcomes are available regardless of adherence to protocol, then an intention to treat analysis is possible. This analysis is one of the "mainstays" of research in which mortality is an important outcome, and it is desirable to estimate the net effect of starting with a treatment assignment. Proponents of the "pragmatic" approach to clinical research tend to favor this method. I believe that psychopharmacologic researchers should consider "unlinking" measurement from compliance to protocol, leaving the option of analyzing all outcomes based on the original randomization group, but this is usually not done in current designs of clinical trials of psychopharmacology.
3. At least some postrandomization information is available on nearly all patients, so that not all dropout occurs right away. If this is not the case, there is very little one can do, as all methods rely on some partial information about the "trajectory" of patients in the study.

As always, which route to take depends on where you want to go. A coherent analysis of clinical trial data that have substantial gaps begins with a clear statement of the aim of the analysis, usually stated in terms of some population parameter. Here are four possible targets of estimation:

1. Patient acceptability of the treatment: Under all circumstances one has available the "completed protocol" indicator itself; if failure to complete (for any reason) is considered a sensible outcome variable, it can be analyzed as a dichotomous outcome. Time to dropout can be analyzed with survival methods. This approach "defines away" the problem of dropout, by making it into an informative outcome.
2. The average last reported value of a response variable ("endpoint analysis"): This method also "defines away" the problem.
3. The mean actual response in all patients in the group, regardless of their protocol status (intent to treat): This approach is not supported by current

patterns of experimentation in psychopharmacology since one does not usually get to measure response in dropouts. Nevertheless, this would be measurable if (as discussed above) the measurement and protocol status were not linked. As long as this is considered a useful summary of response, it also "defines away" the problem of dropout.

4. The mean hypothetical response that would have been observed had all patients remained on the assigned treatment (potential response): This unobserved (and unobservable!) statistic is almost surely at the base of scientific inquiry into the effect of treatment. It is what the investigator would ask for in the best of all possible worlds, and it is what would be estimated if human patients were rats, guinea pigs, or electrons, without choice in the matter of compliance. It is the answer to the patient's question: "What can I expect if I take this medicine?" But it is not observable.

A great deal of confusion results from the fact that the second target of estimation ("endpoint") mentioned above wears another hat: it is sometimes regarded as an estimator of the last target of estimation above (potential response). In this role it is given the title "last value carried forward" (LVCF), to indicate that it is a device for imputation of response to the end of the trial rather than a self-defining outcome. Since any statistic is an unbiased estimator of its expectation (by definition of bias!), as long as the "endpoint" statistics are estimating themselves (in the population) all is well. This property does not necessarily carry over to the LVCF as an estimator of the potential response, as discussed later in this chapter.

It is clear that target 1 is a minimal aim: one should certainly report analyses of adherence. Target 3 is more controversial, but has merits as a summary of the pragmatic effect of starting with the treatment under study. Target 2 (endpoint) is the current "standard" analysis, sometimes in slightly altered form, or restricted to times before dropout exceeds some arbitrary fraction (the famous 70/30 rule). However, some would argue that the endpoint analysis (like analysis of completion) "mixes" too many different outcomes together; the interpretation of the "endpoint" is likely to depend heavily on the details of the experiment, such as its designed final measurement time. It is also hard to deal with the consequences of comparisons between groups that effectively choose different times for the point of comparison, due to different patterns of dropout in time. It may weight early acceptability overmuch, and penalize treatments that are slow to act. One characterization of this approach is that the vagaries of nonresponse determine the target of estimation. But as long as the investigator is willing to let the patient take charge of the measurement process by determining the actual target of estimation, there is no difficulty with this approach.

In contrast, if one is interested in knowing something about the value one would have observed had the patient remained on study and on protocol, then one has a particular population value in mind and one seeks to estimate it with a statistic, with desirable properties like unbiasedness and efficiency. In this effort, any summary based on the LVCF stands at the start on the same footing as other statistical estimators, competes as a putative estimator of the same thing, and can be judged in principle by the same criteria. In this spirit we discuss conditions for one desirable quality, lack of bias, for the mean LVCF, as an estimator of the mean potential response.

The mean LVCF in a treatment group will be an unbiased estimator of the population value of the hypothetical experiment in which all patients adhere to treatment and are available for measurement at the end of the study if there is on average no trend in any sequence of values beginning with the last predrop measure and ending with the designed final measurement. This means, among other things, that the "regression to the mean" and other "nonspecific" trend-forming effects (including spontaneous remission) are nil. Many simple but plausible mechanisms for generating missing data do not support this assumption. For example, if the correlation between subsequent measurements is not perfect, the time trend is not toward worsening, and dropout is determined (perhaps stochastically) by extreme (poor) initial or intermediate response, then the LVCF will be pessimistic by an amount that depends on the balance between the underlying trend in means, the correlation of serial measurements, and the linkage between dropout and outcome. As an imputation strategy, the LVCF has defects that are hard to quantify. Detailed treatment of this issue would take us far beyond the scope of the chapter.

## 12 What Are the Alternative Estimators of the Potential Response?

The analysis of "complete" cases is the simplest and most common approach, but depends on an equally implausible assumption, namely that the dropout data are missing completely at random (MCAR; Little and Rubin 1987). This approach regards the observed sample as a random subsample from the hypothetical complete data set. This has been criticized as naive, misleading, and biased. It is clear that patients who remain on study are likely to have been more satisfied with the effects of treatment, and in my experience, they are nearly always better off on most measures than dropouts (at comparable predrop measurement occasions. Nevertheless, this method offers a place to start to seek improved estimators. If the observed responses (the partial trajectories) are sufficient to define a stratification of the patient group with the property that given the trajectory, dropout and potential response are independent (ignorable nonadherence), then efficient methods are available to produce unbiased estimates of mean potential response (Little and Rubin 1987). To the extent that this assumption is only partially true, the methods will reduce but not eliminate bias.

A subtle version of completer analysis uses a dichotomous variable, such as "recovery," and regards dropout before recovery as a censoring variable. The resulting data are analyzed as "failure-time" measurements, with survival methods (life-table, Kaplan-Meier product-limit estimate, etc.). Although this seems to avoid the problem of dropout, it actually needs a strong (and unlikely) assumption, concerning the expected (hypothetical) future course of the patients who drop while still ill (had he or she remained on treatment): this must be the same as the future course of ill patients who did not drop. But the patients who drop may be "different" than patients who do not drop, even though they are all still ill at some point. Furthermore, this strategy makes most sense when the "recovery" is demonstrably stable, so that patients who recover and then drop must be assumed to have remained well. This is also unlikely.

## 13 Methods Based on Ignorable Nonadherence

The "weakest" assumption that supports unbiased methods of estimation is that given the entire history of the patient up to some point, the probability of remaining on study is independent of the possibly unobservable response of the patient had they remained on study. This assumption is called (by Rubin) MAR, to distinguish it from the stronger MCAR. From this assumption it is possible to construct unbiased estimators that make efficient use of the information in the "trajectories" of the patients observed before dropout. The assumption of "ignorable assignment" links this problem to the large and growing body of work on statistical methods with missing data, summarized in the important work by Little and Rubin (1987). These methods require much more statistical input and computer work, and are somewhat technical, but they also offer a framework for coherent investigation of the consequences of failure of the assumptions, and correctly adjust for the extra uncertainty generated by the missing data. In particular, if the assumption of (conditionally) ignorable dropout is not trustworthy, the prevailing opinion in the field is that a variety of alternative estimates must be provided in a thorough investigation of the effects of different kinds and magnitude of residual association between dropout and potential response. As long as protocols are designed in such a way as to make nonadherence a common outcome, such efforts in the analysis of trials will be necessary in order to achieve valid statistical analyses. Perhaps confrontation with the true extra uncertainty associated with the need to model the process of dropout will encourage researchers to search for designs that are less prone to nonadherence problems, and therefore can be analyzed correctly and with confidence using simpler methods.

## References

Fleiss JL (1986) The design and analysis of clinical experiments. Wiley, New York

Gelenberg AJ, Kane JM, Keller MB, Lavori P, Rosenbaum JF, Cole K, Lavelle J (1989) Comparison of standard and low serum levels of lithium for maintenance treatment of bipolar disorder. N Engl J Med 321:1489–1493

Gilbert J, McPeek B, Mosteller F (1977) Progress in surgery and anesthesia: benefits and risks of innovative therapy. In: Bunker JP, Barnes BA, Mosteller F (eds) The costs, risks, and benefits of surgery. Oxford University Press, New York, pp 124–169

Little RA, Rubin DB (1987) Statistical analysis with missing data. Wiley, New York, 1987

Parloff M (1986) Placebo controls in psychotherapy research: a sine qua non or a placebo for research problems. J Consulting Clin Psychol 54:79–87

# Measuring the Efficacy of Psychotropic Drugs: Clinical Symptoms and Rating Scales

W. MAIER[1] and P. BECH[2]

## 1 Introduction

The pathophysiology of anxiety, affective and schizophrenic disorders is not known. Therefore the efficacy of psychotropic drugs cannot be tested by their effect on the pathophysiology of mental disorders. The efficacy of psychotropic drugs in the treatment of acute episodes can only be evidenced by the reduction of indicators of the severity of the target symptomatology in the controlled drug trials.

The target symptomatology is usually defined in psychopathological terms: the scope of the target symptomatology intended to be treated by the drug under study is identical, or at least similar, to the characteristics of the disorder the patient is suffering from; mental disorders are defined mainly by their psychopathology; sometimes the degree of psychosocial impairment is also a diagnostic criterion. Consequently, the measures of the severity to be reduced by treatment are defined by psychopathological and psychosocial items. These outcome measures are representing the severity (frequency and/or intensity) of clinical symptoms which are characteristic for the disorder to be treated.

Some disorders are defined only by a single clinical symptom. For example, panic disorder is defined by panic attacks; in this case, the intensity or the frequency of panic attacks may serve as the outcome measure in clinical trials. The majority of the disorders are defined by a more complex symptom pattern (e.g. depression is defined by depressed mood associated by sleep and appetite disturbances, psychomotor disturbances and other symptoms often occurring with depressed mood); rating scales composed by a series of items, each of which refers to a particular symptom of depression, are usually applied in testing the efficacy of treatments in these disorders.

Another manner of measuring drug effects is to use global scales (Likert scales); the severity of the disorder or of the degree of impairment is to be rated by only one global assessment. Equally, it is possible to measure the global change during the treatment (relative to baseline) by a global scale. This kind of measurement may apply in all mental disorders.

[1] Psychiatrische Klinik der Universität Mainz, Untere Zahlbacher Str. 8, 6500 Mainz, FRG
[2] Frederiksborg Amts Centralsygehus, 48, Dyrehavevej, 3400 Hillerød, Denmark

Methodology of the Evaluation of Psychotropic Drugs
Editors: O. Benkert, W. Maier, and K. Rickels
(Psychopharmacology Series 8)
© Springer-Verlag Berlin Heidelberg 1990

Two kinds of psychopathological assessments are available for the majority of areas of symptomatology: ratings by the physician (observer rating scales) or by the patient (self-rating scales). Even if both rating procedures refer to the same scope of symptomatology, they reveal different things. Patients usually have a different interpretation of the content of corresponding items than physicians (Kearns et al. 1982).

Measurements based on psychopathological and psychosocial variables are the topic of psychometric theory. Psychometric theory is based on two major concepts: reliability and validity (Nunnally 1978). Against this background the assessment systems of the severity of different disorders and of the outcome measures of drug trials will be reviewed.

## 2 Reliability

Reliability is the indicator of precision of a measurement; precision means reproducibility under identical conditions. A series of factors may contribute to incomplete reliability:

a) Variance due to different raters (rater variance).
b) Variance due to different methods of exploring the patient (information variance).
c) Variance due to different interview situations (situation variance).
d) Variance due to imprecise definitions of the items to be rated (criterion variance).

Whereas all four factors influence the reliability of observer rating scales, only the situation variance contributes to the reliability of self-rating scales. The rater variance in observer scales can be reduced by training of the raters extensively. The information variance may be reduced by using structured clinical interviews providing standardized probes for each item to be rated (Williams 1988). The situation variance may be due to a shift of the symptomatology of the patient from rating to rating; this type of unreliability cannot be completely avoided, for the severity assessment is always an assessment of the present state. The criterion variance may be reduced by enhancing the precision in defining the content of an item.

Two different methods of estimating the reliability of observer-rated assessment schedules are commonly used: the joint-rater and the test-retest setting. The joint-rater setting is based on a single interview per patient. Two raters participate and rate the patient independently; the rating of video-taped interviews by different raters is a special kind of joint-rater setting. The test-retest reliability is assessed by comparing the ratings of two independent raters in two different sessions, with a short interval in between. The joint-rater reliability takes into account only the rater variance and the criterion variance; the test-retest reliability takes into account all four kinds of variance. Therefore, the joint-rater reliability can be expected to be lower than the test-retest reliability. The latter type of reliability assessment is a more realistic estimate, because all sources of variance which may occur are included.

The reliability of self-rating scales can only be estimated by asking patients to fill out the scale twice, at different times. As in the case of the test-retest setting for observer rating scales, the interval between the two occasions should be short, in order to reduce the possibility of an objective reduction of the severity of the disorder.

## 3 Validity

The scores of a valid scale are able to discriminate between different states of the variable to be measured. The optimal criterion of validity is the variable to be measured itself. However, the severity of psychopathological variables cannot be observed directly; they are called latent variables. Therefore, indirect criteria of validity are needed. These criteria are oriented on conditions desirable for scales and on hypotheses held to be true for the quality to be measured. Different aspects of validity are usually distinguished.

### 3.1 Content Validity

Content validity means the adequacy with which the scale and its items tap the domain of the latent variable intended to be measured (Nunnally 1978). This type of validity may be assessed by specifying the domain of the entity to be measured (e.g. by reference to psychiatric textbooks) and by matching the content of the items with the domain specified (face validity). A judgement on the face validity of severity scales of psychopathological variables requires the specification of symptoms and features contributing to the severity. This is a controversial issue (see below). The content validity additionally requires a judgement on the carefulness with which the domain of content has been sampled, and formulated into a series of items and placed into a psychometrically sound test (see issues such as consistency, reliability and psychometric issues, discussed below). It is hard to quantify this kind of validity by a coefficient. The correlation between the global score of the scale (summation) and an independent global expert assessment of the entity intended to be measured by the scale may serve as an indicator of content validity (see concurrent validity).

### 3.2 Concurrent Validity

Concurrent validity is a variant of content validity indicating that a measure under study is at least partly in accordance with other hypothesized measures of the same latent variable. Either a global assessment of the severity of the psychopathological variable under study by an expert (psychiatrist or psychologist) or some other well-established scales measuring the same variable may serve as a yardstick for concurrent validity. In any case, the alternative measures and the scale to be validated should be rated independently. A correlation coefficient between both measures higher than .7 indicates a satisfactory concurrent validity.

### 3.3 Sensitivity to Change

A special aspect of content validity is important for measurements which are used for the assessment of change due to interventions: this is the major field of application for psychiatric severity assessment. The items defining the scale should be sensitive to change. Items describing stable characteristics, such as personality features, are not useful for this purpose. Therefore, judgements on the content validity of psychiatric severity assessments should include an analysis of the sensitivity to change for each of the items.

### 3.4 Construct Validity

Construct validity is crucial for the measurement of all latent variables which cannot be validated by reference to better measures of the variable represented by the scale. Unfortunately, no well-established external (especially biological) indicators of the severity of psychopathological variables are available which can be considered to represent a sound measure of severity. In particular, valid biological indicators of the severity are not available for any psychiatric syndrome, consequently severity assessments in psychiatry have to rely on the construct validity of the scales. A measure for a latent variable has construct validity if:

a) this measure represents a consistent concept – internal construct validity – and
b) this measure behaves as expected (i.e. in accordance with hypotheses on the latent variables which are held to be true) – external construct validity.

Internal construct validity means that the set of items is referring to an underlying variable inducing the correlation between the items (homogeneity, consistency). This underlying variable should remain stable if the scale is applied in different samples (transferability). The global (sum) score of the scale should be able to combine all the information inherent in the items of the scale (sufficiency). Scales with the aforementioned properties define a metric scale: two different individuals may be compared by the global scores of the scale even if they belong to different populations or samples, and even if they have different symptom patterns. A mathematical framework (the Rasch model or more general item-response models) has been developed for testing empirically whether rating data of a scale are in accordance with these properties (Bech 1981; Gibbons et al. 1985). Additionally, latent structure models provide information on the discriminative power of particular items; those models also allow one to identify non optimal scale items (Gibbons et al. 1985).

The major field of application for severity assessment in psychiatry is the assessment of change in drug trials. This field of application provides a special problem for the validity of psychiatric instruments: they should be able to describe change. However, two ratings of the same scale, one at the beginning and the other at the end of the trial, may be inconsistent: side effects occurring during treatment may increase the scores of some items while the scores of other items decrease; the items "depressed mood" and "psychomotor retardation" may have the highest loading when starting the treatment, and the item "sleep disturbances" may have the highest loading at the end of the treatment. In both cases a scale is not measuring the same entity at the beginning and at the end of the treatment. For "cleaning" the scale and for reducing it to a set of consistent items, special psychometric techniques are available, e.g. the dynamic Rasch model (Bech et al. 1986).

The examination of external construct validity is based on generally accepted hypotheses on the variable to be measured. The major hypothesis on the severity of psychopathological variables is that it is reduced by active drugs more than by placebos. Therefore, the most important contribution to the external construct validity of severity assessments comes from placebo-controlled trials also using an active treatment with convincing efficacy: a severity assessment is more valid in this sense the higher the difference in change scores between the placebo and the active treatment group.

Other indicators for external construct validity are derived from diagnostic discriminations between different states of a disease: e.g. endogenous depression (major depressive episodes with melancholia) is usually more severe than dysthymia: this diagnostic discrimination should be reflected by significant differences of global scores on severity scales of depression.

### 3.5 Predictive Validity

This type of validity is crucial if the purpose of the instrument is to estimate some important form of behaviour that is external to the instrument itself, the latter being referred to as the criterion. This type of validity is required if the instrument is used for decision making, e.g. if the severity of the symptomatology is used for deciding between treatments. Predictive validity of severity assessments is important if different levels of severity against a baseline are associated with different contrasts in response to placebo and active treatment, as is the case for pharmacological treatment of depression (Paykel et al. 1988). A coefficient for predictive validity may be the average possible improvement during different treatments for different severity states.

## 4 Other Psychometric Aspects of Reliability and Validity

### 4.1 Internal Consistency

A measure is reliable if it is reproducible on different occasions. The main aspect for psychopathological measurements is their stability across different independent ratings of the same state (test-retest reliability, see above). Another theory of reliability is based on the domain sampling model, which assumes that each scale is a random sample of items from a domain. Parallel measurements are two independent samples of items drawn from the same domain, the relationship of parallel measurements being considered to be an indicator of reliability known as internal consistency. Either the two halves of the set of items defining a scale, or an item and the remaining scale, may be considered to be parallel measurements; the split-half coefficient, the alpha coefficient (Cohen) or the Kuder-Richardson formula 20 (for dichotomous items) characterize this type of reliability.

### 4.2 Homogeneity by Classical Indicators

Psychiatric rating scales should be based on a homogeneous item pool (see above). The homogeneity of content in a test is manifested in the average correlation among items and the pattern of those correlations. Two major methods of analysing homogeneity are proposed by the classical test theory:

a) The item-total correlation, indicating the contribution of an item to the homogeneity of the scale. The item-total correlation is sometimes used in the construction of scales intended to be homogeneous; a low item-total correlation suggests that this item should be omitted.
b) Factor analysis of the item pool, indicating the heterogeneity of a scale by the number of factors. A homogeneous scale should only describe a general factor.
   Both procedures are based on correlation coefficients, therefore they are dependent on the heterogeneity of the sample investigated and their results may be misleading. More recent analyses of homogeneity are based on the Rasch model, which avoids these fallacies.

Taken together, the major aspects for evaluating psychopathological assessments of drug trials are: inter-rater reliability (test-retest reliability), content validity, internal construct validity (homogeneity and transferability by the Rasch model fitting), sensitivity to change, and the ability to measure change (by consistency across different time points evidenced by the dynamic Rasch model analysis).

## 5 Observer Vs Self-Rating Procedures

The evaluation of the efficiency of psychotropic drugs is mainly based on observer-rated assessments (Angst et al. 1989). This convention is justified by the following advantages:

1. Observer rating scales can be applied universally. Severely ill patients often are not able to rate themselves; however, ratings by an interviewer may also be invalid for severe states of the disorder, because patients may be incapable of giving meaningful answers.
2. Observer rating scales are more sensitive than self-rating scales in drug trials. Observer rating scales are especially sensitive for detecting differences of efficacy between placebo and active treatment (Glass et al. 1987).
3. Patient-rated scales usually reveal a higher variance than observer scales. Consequently the sample size necessary for controlling the beta error in controlled drug trials is higher for self-rating than for observer rating scales (Angst et al. 1989).

The advantage of self-rating scales is that they can be applied more frequently (e.g. daily or even more often); observer rating scales are not able to record short-term (e.g. daily) changes. However, this advantage of self-rating scales is not useful for testing the efficacy of psychotropic drugs because the time frame for evidencing efficacy is 3 weeks or more. Some authors even recommend abandoning self-rating scales for testing the efficacy of drugs (Kearns et al. 1982). Other authors recommend using self-rating scales as a supplement to observer rating scales (Angst et al. 1989). Because of the limited utility of self-rating scales for testing the efficacy of drugs they will not be reviewed in the following sections.

## 6 Global Assessments

Global assessments of the severity of the symptomatology by the treating physician are sometimes considered to be valid indicators of the efficacy of psychotropic drugs (Lipman 1982): the severity of complex syndromes is rated by one assessment on a so-called Likert scale (one dimension with multiple ordered categories). Global assessments may focus on particular syndromes such as depression or anxiety (Lipman 1982) or they may be intended to tap the total psychiatric symptomatology by one assessment (CNCPS 1989). However, different experts may use different concepts of the content of the syndromes and the psychiatric symptomatology, so the reliabilty of item-based rating scales, reducing the variability of concepts by defining the items and the weights of items contributing to the severity, can be expected to be superior to global assessment. In spite of this disadvantage, global severity assessments may be useful if no well-accepted or valid rating scales are available; for example this is the case for new diagnostic categories such as panic disorder (CNCPS 1989).

## 7 Measurement of Various Effects

### 7.1 Measurement of Antidepressant Effects (see Table 1)

Currently the 17-item and 21-item Hamilton Depression Scale (HAMD, Hamilton 1960) are the yardstick for measuring the effect of antidepressants in drug trials. Alternative scales – the Montgomery-Asberg Depression Scale with 10 items (MADRS) and the Bech-Rafaelsen Melancholia Scale with 11 items (BRMES) – have been proposed recently (Montgomery and Asberg 1979; Bech et al. 1986). The three scales have in common that they are based mainly on observations of behaviour and less on interview. Both alternative scales are currently used in some drug trials and their acceptance is increasing (Maier et al. 1988b,c).

The reliability of the global scores of these three scales is adequate, but some items of the HAMD reveal flaws in reliability (Rehm and O'Hara 1985; Maier et al. 1988c). The content validity of the HAMD is questionable in spite of its acceptance: the majority of items contributing to the severity of depression are not core symptoms but only loosely associated symptoms, and the correlation with

**Table 1.** Reliability and validity of rating scales for depression, anxiety, mania, and schizophrenia

| Scales | Reliability | Content validity | Concurrent validity (corr. with global assessment) | Internal construct validity | Sensitivity to change | Dynamic Rasch model fitting |
|---|---|---|---|---|---|---|
| HAMD (21-, 17-item versions) | + | Too hetero-geneous | + (No differentiation between moderate and severe states depression) | No Rasch model fitting | + | ? |
| HAMD (6-item version) | + | + | " | + | ? | + |
| MADRS | + | + | + | Divergent results | Insufficient | ? |
| BRMES | + | + | + | + | + | ? |
| HAMA total scale | + | Too hetero-geneous | Insufficient in panic disorder | No Rasch model fitting for total scale | Insufficient | ? |
| Psychic anxiety subscale | + | Heterogeneous | Insufficient in panic disorder | + | + (For general anxiety) | |
| BRMAS Mania | + | + | + | Not available | + | ? |
| Schizophrenia BPRS (10-item version) | + | + | + | + | + | ? |

+, sufficient; ?, not tested; insufficiencies are directly specified.

a global expert assessment of the severity of depression is therefore relatively low. Additionally, the discriminative power of the HAMD between severe and moderate severity of depression is relatively low (Bech et al. 1981; Maier et al. 1988b).

In contrast to the HAMD, the two concurrent scales focus on the core symptomatology of depression. A consequence of the heterogeneity of the HAMD item pool and the homogeneity of the BRMES and MADRS item pools is that the HAMD fails to reveal internal construct validity, evidenced by Rasch model fitting, whereas the BRMES fits the model (Maier and Philipp 1985b; Bech et al. 1981; Maier et al. 1988b,c); the Rasch model fitting of the MADRS is controversial (Allerup 1986; Maier and Philipp 1985b; Maier et al. 1988c). The discriminative power between different levels of severity of depression is adequate for both the BRMES and the MADRS.

Sensitivity to change is adequate for the global scores of the HAMD and the BRMES. Curiously, the MADRS, developed by selecting items sensitive to change from the CPRS (Perris 1986), is inferior in this respect (Maier et al. 1988b,c). The HAMD is the only rating scale also tested by a dynamic Rasch model analysis for its ability to describe change consistently. The HAMD failed to fit this model.

Bech et al. (1981), have derived a subscale of the HAMD, called the Melancholia Scale (MES), comprising six items: 1, "depressed mood"; 2, "guilt feelings"; 7, "work and social disability"; 8, "retardation"; 9, "psychic anxiety"; and 13, "general somatic complaints", by maximizing the discriminatory power. The MES was able to describe change consistently. This six-item subscale was also in congruence with the Rasch model without losing reliability by its brevity (Maier and Philipp 1985a). Consequently, the HAMD is a rather uneconomical scale, without sufficient validity. Alternative scales should be used in addition to the HAMD in antidepressant drug trials.

As discussed by Hamilton (1988), the MES requires a proper interview for completion, as does HDS. Both scales (HDS and MES) can be completed by the same interview. From an interviewing point of view, there is thus no advantage economically in using a shorter scale like the MES rather than the HDS. However, from a statistical point of view it is essential to use well-defined dimensions.

We recommend the use of the MES as a one-dimensional measurement of depressive states and the use, for instance, of the HDS sleep factor for measurement of sedation, or the HDS appetite factor (gastrointestinal symptoms and weight loss) for measurement of appetite stimulation. These factors can be considered in short-term studies as measurements of wanted antidepressive effects, but in long-term studies as side effects of antidepressive treatment.

## 7.2 Measurement of Anxiolytic Effects (see Table 1)

Previously all aspects of anxiety (generalized anxiety phobic symptoms and generalized anxiety) have been the focus of anxiolytics simultaneously. Therefore, scales tapping all aspects of anxiety (e.g. the Hamilton Anxiety Scale HAMA and the Covi Anxiety Scale) have been used as indicators of the efficacy of anxiolytic drugs (Hamilton 1969; Lipman 1981).

The HAMA has been subjected only to a small number of psychometric analyses (Gjerris et al. 1983; Snaith et al. 1982; Maier et al. 1988a) in samples of patients with anxiety neuroses and depressive disorders. The inter-rater reliability turned out to be high. The content validity of the original HAMA was judged to be insufficient (Snaith et al. 1982). A subset of items has only low discriminative power and is more associated with depression or physical disorders than with anxiety; core features of anxiety, such as panic attacks, are not mentioned in the HAMA. Therefore Snaith et al. (1982) propose a modified version of the HAMA, mainly focussing on psychic anxiety and panic attacks. This revised version reveals an increased content validity, evidenced by a higher correlation with the global assessment of severity of anxiety. Beyond this lack of specificity, the HAMA turned out to be too heterogeneous to meet the criteria for internal construct validity; however, the subscale of psychic anxiety did fit the Rasch model. The sensitivity to change of the total score was low (Maier et al. 1988a), because the items describing somatic anxiety were affected by side effects. The subscale of psychic anxiety turned out to be sufficiently sensitive to change. Altogether, the complete HAMA is not able to represent the classical concept of anxiety, and the subscale for psychic anxiety is a better indicator for the severity of anxiety states. However, neither the complete HAMA nor its subscales are able to handle the symptomatology associated with panic attacks.

Recent developments in the conceptualization of anxiety disorders claim that panic disorder, phobic disorders and generalized anxiety disorder are separate diagnostic categories (American Psychiatric Association 1987). Response to treatment is different in these three categories, according to a series of studies. Therefore, testing anxiolytic drugs for their efficacy requires special outcome assessments for each of these three dimensions of anxiety. Special scales for the severity of panic attacks and of phobias are not available. The HAMA subscale of psychic anxiety may serve as an indicator of the severity of generalized anxiety; however, no special validated scales for phobias and panic disorder are available. Therefore the number of panic attacks and a global assessment of the intensity of phobic avoidance are preliminarily used as indicators of severity (CNCPS 1989). The assessment of the efficacy of anxiolytic drugs is therefore blurred by the lack of valid indicators of the severity of anxiety disorders. New scales need to be developed in this field.

### 7.3 Measurement of Antimanic Effects (see Table 1)

Although it is generally agreed that manic states are a clinically more distinct dimension than depression, no specific mania rating scale, analogous to the Hamilton scale for depression, has been included in the first handbooks of psychiatric rating scales (Lyerly and Abbott 1964; Guy 1976).

Hamilton (1988) has argued that because mania is relatively uncommon compared with depression, the construction of mania scales has aroused relatively little interest. He selected (Hamilton 1988) in his review of the assessment of depression and mania the following observer rating scales for mania: the manic state rating scale (Beigel et al. 1971), the modified manic state scale (Blackburn et al. 1977) and the Bech-Rafaelsen Mania Scale (BRMAS, Bech et al. 1978). Whereas the first two scales are designed to be administered by nursing staff covering the entire period (8 h) of a nursing shift, BRMAS is designed to be based on an interview, like the Hamilton or the Melancholia Scales. It seems that the Beigel scale and the BRMAS are still among the most frequently used scales for measurement of antimanic effects.

The inter-observer reliability of the Beigel scale (26 items) and the BRMAS (11 items) is adequate (Bech et al. 1975, 1979). The BRMAS is developed from the Beigel scale including the items that most validly correlated to a global clinical assessment of severity of manic states (Bech et al. 1975). The internal consistency of the BRMAS in terms of intercorrelations of the 11 items has been found acceptable (Bech et al. 1979).

When comparing different antimanic treatments, Shopin et al. (1975) found that the Brief Psychiatric Rating Scale (BPRS; Overall and Gorham 1962) was too insensitive as an outcome measurement. In a recent study (Small et al. 1988), in which the antimanic effects of electroconvulsive therapy (ECT) and lithium were compared, it was found that the MAS was more sensitive than the BPRS in measuring changes in manic states.

So far a penetrating Rasch analysis of the BRMAS is lacking. In a preliminary analysis of the hierarchy of manic items on the MAS it has been found that increased mood level, verbal activity and intrusiveness were among the mild to moderate symptoms, whereas increased self esteem, hostility and increased sexual interest were among the moderate to severe symptoms of mania.

This is in harmony with the study of Young et al. (1983), who made a latent class analysis of five mania items that are all included in the BRMAS. The hierarchical order of these five items was: manic mood, increased motor activity, increased verbal activity, increased self-esteem, and flight of ideas (Young et al. 1983).

In a study on haloperidol plasma levels in relation to antimanic effect it was shown that a concentration of around 4 ng haloperidol/ml plasma gave the best score reduction on the BRMAS (Gjerris et al. 1980).

In long-term studies of manic-depressive patients it is often relevant to measure both depressive and manic mood swings. An index of morbidity should include, for instance, the combined use of Melancholia and Mania Scales (Rafaelsen et al. 1980).

## 7.4 Measurement of Antipsychotic Effects

Of the three rating scales for measuring changes in states of psychotic patients during treatment that were included in the *Handbook of Psychiatric Rating Scales* (Lyerly and Abbott 1964) the BPRS (Overall and Gorham 1962) was the only scale that has survived. In principle, BPRS is a second generation scale as it has been derived from the very comprehensive Lorr Multidimensional Scale for Rating Psychiatric Patients (Lorr 1953).

It was shown that the 16 items of the original BPRS were the most sensitive items for assessing the antipsychotic effect of neuroleptics in schizophrenic patients. The global (total) score of these items was therefore recommended as a sufficient measurement of antipsychotic effects. The inter-observer reliability was found adequate (Lyerly and Abbott 1964). The concurrent validity of the BPRS, when compared to the Lorr scale, was found to be high (0.94). The BPRS has later been enlarged from 16 to 18 items in an attempt to cover other psychopathological states than schizophrenia (Overall 1979).

It seems, however, that the 18-item BPRS has as its main objective the measurement of schizophrenic or schizo-affective states. A detailed review of the literature on the 18-item BPRS with its reliability in different cultures has been published by Hedlund and Vieweg (1980).

A 10-item BPRS subscale for schizophrenia has been suggested by Overall (1979), but the validity and reliability of this scale has only recently been analysed (Bech et al. 1989; Andersen et al. 1989).

Although other scales have been developed for the measurement of antipsychotic effects (e.g. Montgomery et al. 1978; Manchanda et al. 1986) the content validity of the new scales does not differ from BPRS. The advantage of the new scales are anchoring definitions of each item, since one of the weakness of the original BPRS was lack of proper item definition. A BPRS version with five-point item definitions, analogous to HDS, has been developed by Bech et al. (1986). The psychometric aspects of the 10-item BPRS subscale for schizophrenia with the five-point item definition have been analysed by Andersen et al. (1989) who found the interobserver reliability adequate. It was furthermore demonstrated that these ten items had an additive relation, since they fulfilled the Rasch model. As discussed elsewhere (Bech 1986), the following three BPRS items can be considered as negative symptoms of schizophrenia: blunted or inappropriate affect, conceptual disorganization and emotional withdrawal. The remaining six BPRS items can be considered as positive symptoms of schizophrenia: suspiciousness, hallucinations, exaggerated self-esteem, hostility, uncooperativeness, and unusual thought content, whereas the item of specific motor disturbances is best considered separately in the context of negative and positive symptoms of schizophrenia. This subdivision of the ten BPRS items of schizophrenia is largely in harmony with the Rasch analysis performed by Levine et al. (1983) who used the Schedule for Affective Disorders and Schizophrenia as the assessment system. The Rasch analysis of the BPRS subscale by Andersen et al. (1989) has indicated the adequacy of having only one dimension of severity of schizophrenic states upon which the negative and positive symptoms can be listed.

As discussed by Wing (1987), most schizophrenic disorders tend to be characterized by both negative and positive symptoms. The three BPRS items of negative symptoms: blunted affect, conceptual disorganization and emotional withdrawal, were selected by Overall and Gorham (1962) because these items still seemed to improve during antipsychotic treatment. The Rasch analysis has confirmed the additive relationship between these three negative symptoms and the remaining positive symptoms included in the BPRS subscale of schizophrenia. Additionally rating scales have recently been designed that selectively focus on negative and positive symptoms of schizophrenia (e.g. Andreasen and

Olsen 1982; Kay et al. 1986). The sensitivity of these scales for the measurement of antipsychotic effects is still under investigation. At this moment it seems justified to conclude that the BPRS subscale of schizophrenia is a short and relevant rating scale for measuring the outcome of treatments of patients with psychoses of schizophrenia or a related nature.

### 7.5 Measurement of the Efficacy of Long-Term (Prophylactic) Treatment

The long-term treatment of psychotropic drugs is oriented at other outcome criteria than short-term acute treatment. The two major aims of long-term treatment are:

a) Prophylactic treatment after full or partial remission.
b) Treatment of chronic patients, i.e. subjects not remitting during short-term treatment.

Prophylactic treatment is mainly focussed on the prevention of new episodes of the disorder after a remission following one episode or a series of episodes. One main outcome measure is consequently the duration of the period without a new episode. The definition of the beginning of an episode is crucial for this outcome measure. However, this is a controversial issue: different conventions for defining the beginning and the end of major depressive episodes have been established (Keller and Shapiro 1982; Prien et al. 1984; Prien and Kupfer 1986). Extra treatment required during the long-term trials is also used as an indicator of the efficacy (Coppen et al. 1978).

No generally accepted proposal for the beginning and the end of psychotic disorders is available up to now. Because of the apparent difficulties in defining the beginning and the end of schizophrenic episodes, the efficacy of prophylactic treatment in schizophrenia and related disorders is usually measured by the time interval to the next admission to hospital after discharge, or the number or duration of hospitalisations during long-term treatment. Additionally, extra treatment required during the trial is used as an indicator of efficacy (Carpenter et al. 1987).

The evaluation of long-term treatment relies in addition on the cross-sectional or longitudinal retrospective assessment of psychosocial impairment and functioning, and on the quality of life assessment (Bradley and Hirsch 1986; Carpenter et al. 1987; see also the chapter by Bech, this volume). A series of scales has been proposed for this purpose (Bradley and Hirsch 1987; Carpenter et al. 1987; Bech 1989). Generally, these scales are less well validated than the psychopathological rating scales (Bradley and Hirsch 1986).

## 8 Conclusion

In the absence of external indicators of the severity of syndromes, the measurement of the efficacy of psychotropic drugs must rely on the assessment of psychopathological symptomatology using rating scales or on the important symptoms. This review has demonstrated that the rating scale procedures currently used in measuring the efficacy of psychotropic drugs are by no means perfect. In particular, the evaluation of anxiolytic drugs is complicated by the lack of valid rating scale procedures for measuring treatment outcome. The measurement of the efficacy of long-term treatment is also inadequate, as no convention on the major outcome criteria is generally accepted.

## References

Allerup P (1986) Statistical analysis of MADRS – a rating scale. The Danish Institute for Educational Research

American Psychiatric Association (1987) DSM-III-R. American Psychiatric Association, Washington

Andersen J, Larsen JK, Schultz V, Nielsen BM, Kizner A, Behnke K, Munk-Anderson, Butler B, Allerup P, Bech P (1989) The brief psychiatric rating scale. Dimension of schizophrenia – reliability and construct validity. Psychopathology (in press)

Andreasen NC, Olsen S (1982) Negative vs positive schizophrenia. Definition and validation. Arch Gen Psychiatry 39:789–794

Angst J, Hippius H, Woggon B (1989) Consensus conference on the methodology of clinical trials in antidepressants. Pharmacopsychiatry 22:3–7

Bech P (1981) Rating scales for affective disorders: their validity and consistency. Acta Psychiatr Scand 64[Suppl 295]:1–101

Bech P (1986) Methods to evaluate depressive and psychotic symptoms. In: Pepplinkhuizen, Verhoeven (eds) Biological psychiatry in Europe today. Uitgeverij, Leiden, pp 55–58

Bech P, Bolwig TG, Dein E, Jacobsen O, Gram LF (1975) Quantitative Rating of Manic States. Acta Psychiatr Scand 52:1–6

Bech P, Rafaelsen OJ, Kramp P, Bolwig TG (1978) The mania rating scale: construction and inter-observer agreement. Neuropharmacology 17:430–431

Bech P, Bolwig TG, Kramp P, Rafaelsen OJ (1979) The Bech-Rafaelsen mania scale and the Hamilton depression scale. Acta Psychiatr Scand 59:420–430

Bech P, Allerup P, Gram L, Reisby N, Rosenberg R, Jacobsen D, Nagy A (1981) The Hamilton rating scale: evaluation of objectivity using logistic models. Acta Psychiatr Scand 63:290–299

Bech P, Kastrup M, Rafaelsen OJ (1986) Minicompendium of rating scales for anxiety, depression, mania, schizophrenia with corresponding DSM-III syndromes. Acta Psychiatr Scand 73[Suppl 326]:1–37

Beigel A, Murphy DL, Bunney WE (1971) The manic-state rating scale. Arch Gen Psychiatry 25:256–262

Blackburn IM, London JB, Ashworth CM (1977) A new scale for measuring mania. Psychol Med 7:453–458

Bradley PB, Hirsch SR (1986) The psychopharmacology and treatment of schizophrenia. British Association for Psychopharmacology, Monograph no 8. Oxford Medical, Oxford

Carpenter WT Jr, Heinrichs DW, Hanlon TE (1987) A comparative trial of pharmacologic strategies in schizophrenia. Am J Psychiatry 144:1466–1470

Coppen A, Ghose K, Montgomery S, Rama Rao VA, Bailey J, Jorgensen A (1978) Continuation therapy with amitriptyline in depression. Br J Psychiatry 133:28–33

Gibbons RD, Clark DC, von Ammon Cavanaugh S, Davis JM (1985) Application of modern psychometric theory in psychiatry research. J Psychiatr Res 19:43–55

Gjerris A, Bech P, Broen-Christensen C, Geisler A, Klysner R, Rafaelsen OJ (1980) Haloperidol plasma levels in relation to antimanic effect. In: Usdin E, Dahl S, Gram LF, Lingjaerde O (eds) Clinical pharmacology and psychiatry. MacMillan, London

Gjerris A, Bech P, Bojholm S, Bowlig TG, Kramp P, Clemmensen L, Andersen J, Jensen E, Rafaelsen OJ (1983) The Hamilton Anxiety Scale. Evaluation of homogeneity and inter-observer reliability in patients with depressive disorders. J Affect Disord 5:163–170

Glass RM, Uhlenhuth EH, Kellner R (1987) The value of self-report assessment in studies of anxiety disorders. J Clin Psychopharmacol 7(4):215–221
Guy W (1976) Early clinical drug evaluation (ECDEU) assessment manual for psychopharmacology. National Institute of Mental Health, Rockville (publ no 76-338)
Hamilton M (1960) A rating scale for depression. J Neurosurg Psychiatry 23:56–62
Hamilton A (1969) Diagnosis and rating of anxiety. Br J Psychiatry Special Publication no 3:76–79
Hamilton M (1988) Assessment of depression and mania. In: Georgotas A, Cancro R (eds) Depression and mania. Elsevier, New York, pp 625–637
Hedlund JL, Vieweg BW (1980) The Brief Psychiatric Rating Scale (BPRS): a comprehensive review. J Operational Psychiatry 11:48–65
Kay SR, Opler LA, Fiszbein A (1986) Positive and negative syndrome scale (PANSS) rating manual. Department of Psychiatry, Albert Einstein College of Medicine, New York
Kearns NP, Cruickshank CA, McGuigan K, Rilag SA, Shaw SP, Snaith RP (1982) A comparison of depression rating scales. Br J Psychiatry 141:45–49
Keller MB, Shapiro RW (1982) "Double depression": superimposition of acute depressive episodes on chronic depressive disorders. Am J Psychiatry 139:438–442
Lewine RJ, Fogg L, Meltzer HY (1983) Assessment of negative and positive symptoms in schizophrenia. Schizophrenia Bull 9:368–376
Lipman RS (1982) Differentiating anxiety and depression in anxiety disorders: use of rating scales. Psychopharmacol Bull 18:69–82
Lorr M (1953) Multidimensional scale for rating psychiatric patients. Vet Admin Technol Bull 43:10–507
Lyerly SB, Abbott PS (1964) Handbook of psychiatric rating scales. National Institute of Mental Health, Bethesda
Maier W, Philipp M (1985a) Comparative analysis of observer depression scales. Acta Psychiatr Scand 72:239–245
Maier W, Philipp M (1985b) Improving the assessment of severity of depressive states: a reduction of the Hamilton Depression Scale. Pharmacopsychiatry 18:114–115
Maier W, Buller R, Philipp M, Heuser I (1988a) The Hamilton anxiety scale: reliability, validity and sensitivity to change in anxiety and depressive disorders. J Affective Disord 14:61–68
Maier W, Heuser I, Philipp M, Frommberger U, Demuth W (1988b) Improving depression severity assessment. II. Content, concurrent and external validity of three observer depression scales. J Psychiatr Res 22(1):13–19
Maier W, Philipp M, Heuser I, Schlegel S, Buller R, Wetzel H (1988c) Improving depression severity assessment. I. Reliability, internal validity and sensitivity to change of three observer depression scales. J Psychiatr Res 22(1):3–12
Manchanda R, Saupe R, Hirsch SR (1986) Comparison between brief psychiatric rating scale and the Manchester scale for the rating of schizophrenic symptoms. Acta Psychiatr Scand 74: 563–568
Montgomery SA, Asberg M (1979) A new depression scale designed to be sensitive to change. Br J Psychiatry 134:382–389
Montgomery SA, Taylor P, Montgomery D (1978) Development of a schizophrenia scale sensitive to change. Neuropharmacology 17:1061–1063
Nunally JC (1978) Psychometric theory. McGraw-Hill, New York
Overall JE (1979) Criteria for the selection of subjects for research in biological psychiatry. In: von Pragh HM, Lader MH, Rafaelsen OJ, Sachar EJ (eds) Handbook of biological psychiatry. Dekker, New York, pp 359–391
Overall JE, Gorham DR (1962) The brief psychiatric rating scale Psychol Rep 10:799–812
Paykel ES, Hollyman JA, Freeling P, Sedgwick P (1988) Predictors of therapeutic benefit from amitriptyline in mild depression: a general practice placebo-controlled trial. J Affective Disord 14:83–95
Perris C (1986) Rating of depression with a subscale of the CPRS. In: Sartorius N, Ban TA (eds) Assessment of depression. Springer, Berlin Heidelberg New York, pp 90–107
Prien RF, Kupfer DJ (1986) Continuation drug therapy for major depressive episodes: how long should it be maintained? Am J Psychiatry 143:18–23

Prien RF, Kupfer DJ, Mansky PA, Small JG, Tuason VB, Voss CB, Johnson WE (1984) Drug therapy in the prevention of recurrences in unipolar and bipolar affective disorders. Arch Gen Psychiatry 41:1096–1104

Rafaelsen OJ, Bech P, Bolwig TG, Kramp P, Gjerris A (1980) The Bech-Rafaelsen combined rating scale for mania and melancholia. Psychiatr Fennica [Suppl]:327–331

Rehm LP, O'Hara MW (1985) Item characteristics of the Hamilton Rating Scale for Depression. J Psychiatry Res 19:31–41

Shopin B, Gershou S, Thompson H, Collins P (1975) Psychoactive drugs in mania. Arch Gen Psychiatry 32:34–42

Small JG, Klapper MH, Kellams JJ, Miller MJ, Milstein V, Sharpley PN, Small IF (1988) Electroconvulsive treatment compared with lithium in the management of manic states. Arch Gen Psychiatry 45:727–732

Snaith RP, Bough SJ, Clayden AD, Husain A, Sipple MA (1982) The Clinical Anxiety Scale: an instrument derived from the Hamilton Anxiety Scale. Br J Psychiatry 141:518–523

Williams JBW (1988) A structured interview guide for the Hamilton depression rating scale. Arch Gen Psychiatry 45:742–747

Wing JK (1987) Psychosocial factors affecting the long-term course of schizophrenia. In: Strauss JS, Bööker W, Brenner HD (eds) Psychosocial treatment of schizophrenia. Huber, Toronto

Young MA, Abrams R, Raylor MA, Meltzer HY (1983) Establishing diagnostic criteria for mania. J Nerv Ment Dis 171:676–682

# Methodological Problems in Assessing Quality of Life as Outcome in Psychopharmacology: A Multiaxial Approach

P. Bech[1]

## 1 Quality of Life Assessed as a Discomfort

Clinical research into quality of life has increased intensively since 1964, when this concept was introduced (Bech 1987a). In medicine, quality of life has been analysed especially in clinical trials of cardiovascular therapies (Wenger et al. 1984) and of cancer treatment (Aaronsen and Beckmann 1986). In psychiatric and psychological research the measurement of quality of life was developed before 1964 under the headings of discomfort (Parloff et al. 1954) or subjective adjustment (Veroff et al. 1962). As discussed elsewhere (Bech 1987a), the concept of discomfort was developed by a group of psychiatrists, who found it important to measure comfort, effectiveness and self-awareness as criteria of improvement in psychotherapy. After pilot studies they concluded:

In choosing measures of comfort it became obvious that since this is a subjective state no one can judge it but the patient. It seemed wise to construct the chief measure of this criterion in terms not of comfort but its opposite – discomfort – since almost all out-patients seek treatment to be relieved of distress, rather than to be helped to move from a satisfactory state of comfort to a better one... (Parloff et al. 1954).

Against this background Parloff and coworkers constructed a self-rating scale including items as shown in Table 1. It is of interest that this questionnaire has been further developed since 1954 and is now one of the most widely used American questionnaires for psychopathology, the Hopkins Symptom Checklist (Derogatis et al. 1974) or the Self-Report Symptom Checklist (SCL-90) (Guy 1976).

## 2 Well-Being Versus Social Functioning

In a later overview, Parloff (1970) separated the dimension of well-being from the dimension of social functioning. Table 2 shows a modified version of Parloff's model. A similar distinction has been made in DSM-III (American Psychiatric Association 1980), where axis 1 reflects the psychic symptomatology and axis 5 the

[1] Frederiksborg General Hospital, Department of Psychiatry, 48, Dyrehavevej, DK-3400 Hillerød

Methodology of the Evaluation of Psychotropic Drugs
Editors: O. Benkert, W. Maier, and K. Rickels
(Psychopharmacology Series 8)
© Springer-Verlag Berlin Heidelberg 1990

**Table 1.** SCL Discomfort Scale: relationship to Eysenck General Neurotic Behaviour

| | Corresponding items | |
|---|---|---|
| | Eysenck and Eysenck (1976) | SCL Derogatis et al. (1974) |
| Blaming yourself for things | 12 | 26 |
| Feeling critical of others | – | 6 |
| Your feelings being easily hurt | 19/80 | 34 |
| Feeling irritable | 15/88 | 11 |
| Feeling hopeless about future | 62 | 54 |
| Feeling blue | 3/7 | 30 |
| Feeling lonely | 77 | 29 |
| Temper outburst | – | 24 |
| Thoughts of ending your life | 68 | 15 |
| Trouble remembering things | – | 9 |
| Having to do things very slowly | 84 | 38 |
| Difficulty making decisions | – | 46 |
| Trouble concentrating | – | 55 |
| Your mind going blank | – | 51 |
| Sexual interests | – | 5 |
| Trouble falling asleep | 54 | 44 |
| Feeling low in energy | 58 | 14 |
| Self-rating discomfort scale | | SCL-17 |

**Table 2.** Dimensions of outcome of treatment

| Quality of life elements | Adjustment | | Mind-expanding | |
|---|---|---|---|---|
| Well-being | Discomfort | | Pleasure | |
| | | Distress | | Joy |
| | | Dissatisfaction | | Love |
| | | Dysphoria | | |
| Social functioning | Ineffective | | Creative | |
| | | Inept | | Energetic |
| | | Incompetent | | Powerful |
| | | Inefficient | | Persuasive |

Modified after Parloff (1970).

social functioning. In contrast, axis 5 in DSM-III-R (American Psychiatric Association 1987) is a mixture of psychic symptoms and social functioning. A divergent validity between the two Parloff dimensions can be seen in the state of cannabis intoxication, during which a psychic experience of happiness might emerge although the social functioning in this state is clearly reduced. One of the co-authors of the original discomfort scale has later preferred the term demoralization to discomfort. Hence, Frank (1974) says that:

"... demoralization describes the state of candidates for psychotherapy, whatever their diagnostic label. They are conscious of having failed to meet their own expectations or those of others, or being unable to cope with some pressing problems. They feel powerless to change the situation or themselves. Their life is constricted both in space and time... the demoralized person is prey to anxiety and depression (the two most common complaints of persons seeking psychotherapy)... ".

The subjective state of demoralization can, according to Frank, be measured as dimensions of anxiety or depression. The extensional (i.e., that items of a scale have an additive relationship to ensure that their total score is a sufficient statistic) concept of quality of life can consequently be measured by items found in the original discomfort scale (Table 1). In our studies in psychosomatic research we have preferred the General Health Questionnaire (Goldberg 1972). In Table 3 is shown a selection of items from the General Health Questionnaire.

**Table 3.** A sample of items of the General Health Questionnaire relevant for measuring quality of life

| Have you recently: | |
|---|---|
| (1) | – being feeling perfectly well and in good health? |
| (7) | – been able to concentrate on whatever you're doing? |
| (16) | – been feeling full of energy? |
| (23) | – tended to lose interest in your ordinary activities? |
| (28) | – felt on the whole you were doing things well? |
| (30) | – been satisfied with the way you've carried out your task? |
| (31) | – been able to feel warmth and affection for those near to you? |
| (35) | – felt that you are playing a useful part in things? |
| (36) | – felt capable to making decisions about things? |
| (42) | – been able to enjoy your normal day to day activities? |
| (54) | – been feeling reasonably happy, all things considered? |

( ) Original item number.

## 3 The Scaling of Subjective Feelings

It is generally accepted that Thurstone (1928) was one of the first who measured attitudes by the use of questionnaires. He had as a psychologist great experience with psychophysics. Inspired by Fechner's Law on subjective discrimination of physical stimuli, Thurstone defined attitudes as the sum total of a man's inclinations and feelings about any specified topic. Thurstone's attitude scales contained the method of paired comparisons which still seemed associated with Fechner's subjective discrimination technique in psychophysics. The Likert (1932) scaling method which simply used item response categories (e.g. "strongly agree", "agree", "uncertain") soon became more popular than the Thurstone method. Both Thurstone and Likert analysed the scaling problems of their attitude scales. Likert made the requirement that the items of an attitude scale should have an additive relationship if the summed total of the scale was a measurement of the attitude under investigation. As the evaluation of the scale's internal consistency Likert used item-total scoare correlations.

Stevens (1962) reformulated Fechner's Law as the so-called power function, which says that in psychophysics the subjective sensory response is closely related to the physical stimulus. The use of visual analogue scales can be considered as a consequence of the work of Stevens and coworkers.

The relationship between visual analogue scales or global scales (Bech et al. 1986) and Likert scales has only been analysed to a limited degree. When comparing the Hamilton Depression Scale (Hamilton 1960) and a global scale for depression, we found a curvilinear relationship (Bech et al. 1975). This result was in harmony with Miller's Law on the amount of transmitted information, indicating that the number of items transmitted by Likert scales is 7 $\pm 2$ (Miller 1956).

Against this background we advocated the use of Rasch item analysis of Likert scales when measuring dimensions of subjective feelings such as depression (Bech 1981). From this, it can be seen that during the last three decades there has been a growing development of scales, global as well as Likert to measure quantitatively states such as discomfort.

## 4 Hedonia Vs Anhedonia: The Problem of Measuring Quality of Life in Psychiatry

The quality of life as measured by well-being or discomfort scales has a logical correspondence to hedonia. Only in persons who believe that the conquest of happiness is a basic human need (i.e. hedonics) is it meaningful to measure degrees of well-being extensionally.

The intensional (i.e., that items of scale have a meaningful reference of validity to ensure that they not only are sufficient but also necessary) aspects of demoralization in psychiatric patients has, as previously mentioned, been described by Frank (1974): "They are conscious of having failed to meet their own expectations or those of others, or being unable to cope with some pressing problems". This subjective concept of morality is seen most markedly in the neurotic personality. Character neurotics can be considered as hedonics with a subnormal state of well-being resulting from an over-concern with the norms of morality. At the other extreme in the large group of hedonics are the psychopathics who are less concerned with the norms of morality, in severe cases termed sociopaths.

The third category of personality disorder in psychiatry (Bech et al. 1987), the borderline personality deviation, includes anhedonics, i.e., persons who have ontological uncertainties about the existence of the goodness of life. Figure 1 shows the intensional items of goodness of life as found in Griffin's monograph (1986). Borderlines have a basic ambivalence about the existence of such items as "deep personal relations".

Scales measuring quality of life extensionally with an intensional relation to elements of goodness of life, as shown in Fig. 1, are not applicable in cases of borderline personality or in schizophrenia. Anhedonia is not equivalent to depression, as discussed elsewhere (Bech 1987b).

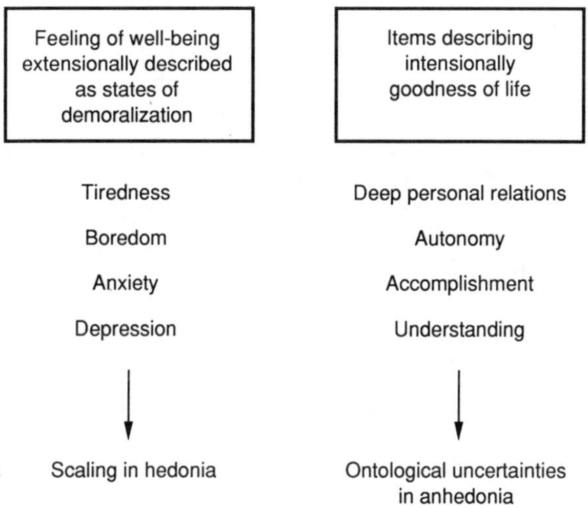


**Fig. 1.** Hedonia vs anhedonia in quality of life

## 5 Discomfort Vs Disability in Schizophrenia

Most scales claiming to measure quality of life are assessing disability rather than discomfort. Hence, one of the most frequently used scales in general medicine, the Nottingham Health Profile (Hunt et al. 1981), is a scale for disability of physical illness and not for discomfort as defined by well-being. Likewise, another frequently used scale for measuring quality of life, the Health Opinion Survey (MacMillan 1957) assesses autonomic hyperactivity, which can be considered as a disability of neurotic behaviour.

The dimensions of disability in schizophrenia have been described as positive and negative syndromes. From a psychometric point of view these two syndromes have been most thoroughly evaluated by Levine et al. (1983). Using the Schedule for Affective Disorders and Schizophrenia (SADS), these authors found that the following items had an additive relationship in schizophrenic patients: blunted affect, conceptual disorganization, emotional withdrawal and slowed body movements. This rank order of negative symptoms fulfilled the Rasch model of dimensional statistics. Furthermore, Levine et al. (1983) found that the following items had an additive relationship: hallucinations, suspiciousness, unusual thought content, and exaggerated self-esteem. This rank order of positive symptoms also fulfilled the Rasch model of dimensional statistics.

In a recent study we evaluated the ten items of the Brief Psychiatric Rating Scale (BPRS) which Overall (1979) found to be the schizophrenia subscale of BPRS. Using a Rasch analysis we found that the negative and positive syndromes as defined by the Levine study (Bech et al. 1988a) statistically are describing one major dimension of severity of schizophrenic states. In other words, the positive syndrome is a necessary but not sufficient part of schizophrenia.

These results are in harmony with the Holden et al. (1971) study on predictor patterns in schizophrenia. The clinical impression scale of schizophrenia (Guy 1976), which is a global severity scale, was found to be the most meaningful scale when predicting outcome in schizophrenia.

In some studies the non-schizophrenic items of BPRS (e.g. anxiety, guilt and depressed mood) have been used to evaluate quality of life in schizophrenia. Because schizophrenic patients in principle are anhedonics, it is very difficult to apply a well-being scale. Schizophrenic illness gives so profound a disability that studies in this field should be most concerned about using a valid dimension of disability in combination with a valid scale for side effects. We recommend the use of a global clinical assessment of severity of schizophrenic states, the ten item BPRS subscale for schizophrenia, and the UKU side effect scale (Lingjærde et al. 1987).

## 6 Discomfort Vs Disability in Depression

The nosology of depression is more clearly defined than the many descriptive terms of melancholia indicates. At the phenomenological level depression can be classified as minor and major with reference to severity (Bech et al. 1984). Diagnostically, depression can be classified as endogenous, reactive and mixed endogenous-reactive (Bech et al. 1988b). Minor reactive depression is often called neurotic depression. Both neurotics and patients with manic-depressive disorders are hedonics. Outside the depressive episodes these patients are highly productive persons and it is very important to evaluate quality of life in recurrent depressive disorders.

As discussed elsewhere (Bech 1988), scales measuring side effects of antidepressants or lithium can be termed distress scales, in contrast to discomfort scales which have a psychometric transparency to attitude of illness. The self-rating scale developed on the basis of the Beck Depression Inventory, the symptom rating scale for depression and anxiety, includes both side effect items and items for asthenia, anxiety and depression (Bech and Hey 1979). In conclusion, when measuring disability of depression we recommend the use of observer rating scales such as the Hamilton-Melancholic Scale. When measuring distress or discomfort the General Health Questionnaire or the symptom rating scale for asthenia, anxiety and depression are relevant scales.

## 7 Discomfort in Non-Disabled Patients

Patients with mild hypertension have no disability, hence the term "asymptomatic" hypertension. In a study on 303 patients with mild hypertension (Bech et al. 1990) we measured the subjective state of quality of life both by use of visual analogue scales and by use of the General Health Questionnaire. Psychosocial stressors were measured by Holmes and Rahe's (1967) social readjustment rating scale.

The results showed that 36% of the patients were cases of discomfort, according to Goldberg's cut-off or threshold score on the General Health Questionnaire for being non-normal. Applying a multiple regression analysis of "caseness" (normals versus cases) of discomfort over the variables age, sex, treatment, side effects, blood pressure and life events, we found that life events and side effects accounted significantly for the variance of caseness.

Furthermore, we found a linear relationship between the General Health Questionnaire and the visual analogue scale measuring well-being "all things considered". The results of this study confirm the strategy (Bech 1987a) that it is important to use a multiaxial approach of quality of life in psychosomatic research.

## 8 Conclusion

The concept of quality of life was originally measured as degrees of discomfort in patients seeking psychotherapy. The discomfort scale is, like the General Health Questionnaire (Table 3), a scale measuring subjective well-being. In a multiaxial approach to quality of life these scales can be considered as axis 1 (psychic symptoms) which might be distinguished from axis 5 (social functioning).

From a psychometric point of view the discomfort questionnaires fulfil the criteria of scaling subjective feelings. However, these scales have a logical correspondence to hedonia. Only in persons who believe that the conquest of happiness is a basic human need (hedonics) is it meaningful to measure degrees of well-being on a scale. In other words, personality disorders (axis 2) are an important axis to take into account in quality of life measurements.

Borderline personalities and schizophrenics are anhedonics, i.e. these persons have ontological uncertainties about the goodness of life. Their ambivalence towards the existence of the items shows in Fig. 1 means that discomfort scales are not applicable in this personality category.

Most scales claiming to measure quality of life are assessing disability (the clinical symptoms of the disease) rather than discomfort (well-being), e.g. the Nottingham Health Profile which measures physical disability. In schizophrenia, disabilities have been described as positive and negative syndromes. Psychometrically, however, it has been shown that these syndromes are describing only one dimension, severity of illness. Disability and side effects of treatment are, therefore, the dimensions most relevant when measuring outcome in schizophrenia.

In depression, observer rating scales like the Hamilton Depression Scale and the Melancholia Scale are the relevant scales for measuring disability. When measuring discomfort, questionnaires like the General Health Questionnaire or the modified Beck Depression Inventory (which includes subscales for anxiety, asthenia and side effects) or the SCL-90 are recommended.

In non-disabled patients such as patients with "asymptomatic" hypertension it has been shown that cases of discomfort can be explained by side effects to treatment and/or life events. Psychosocial stressors (axis 4) are, therefore, an important axis to take into account in quality of life measurements.

In conclusion, the multiaxial approach involving all five DSM-III axes is necessary when measuring quality of life in psychopharmacology. As an extra axis in this respect, side effects of treatment must be included.

## References

Aaronsen NK, Beckmann J (eds) (1986) The quality of life of cancer patients. Raven, New York

American Psychiatric Association (1980) Diagnostic and statistical manual of mental disorders, 3rd edn. (DSM-III). American Psychiatric Association, Washington DC

American Psychiatric Association (1987) Diagnostic and statistical manual of mental disorders, 3rd rev edn. (DSM-III-R). American Psychiatric Association, Washington DC

Bech P (1981) Rating scales for affective disorders. Their validity and consistency. Acta Psychiatr Scand 64 [Suppl 295]:1-101

Bech P (1987a) Quality of life in psychosomatic research. Psychopathology 20:169-179

Bech P (1987b) Concept of mild endogenous depression. Br J Psychiatry 151:271

Bech P (1988) Rating scales for mood disorders: applicability, consistency and construct validity. Acta Psychiatr Scand 78 [Suppl 345]:45-55

Bech P, Hey H (1979) Depression or asthenia related to metabolic disturbances in obese patients after intestinal by-pass surgery. Acta Psychiatr Scand 59:462-470

Bech P, Gram LF, Dein E, Jacobsen O, Vitger J, Bolwig TG (1975) Quantitative rating of depressive states. Acta Psychiatr Scand 51:161-170

Bech P, Allerup P, Reisby N, Gram LF (1984) Assessment of symptom change from improvement curves on the Hamilton depression scale in trials with antidepressants. Psychopharmacology 84:276-281

Bech P, Kastrup M, Rafaelsen OJ (1986) Minicompendium for rating scales. Acta Psychiatr Scand 73 [Suppl 326]:1-37

Bech P, Hjortsø S, Lund K, Vilmar T, Kastrup M (1987) An integration of the DSM-III and ICD-8 by global severity assessments for measuring multidimensional outcomes in general hospital psychiatry. Acta Psychiatr Scand 75:297-306

Bech P, Larsen JK, Andersen J (1988a) The BPRS: psychometric developments. Psychopharmacol Bull 24:118-121

Bech P, Allerup P, Gram LF, Kragh-Sørensen P, Rafaelsen OJ, Reisby N, Vestergaard P, Danish University Antidepressant Group (DUAG) (1988b) The diagnostic melancholia scale (DMS): dimensions of endogenous and reactive depression with relationship to the Newcastle scales. J Affective Disord 14:161–170

Bech P, Loldrup D, Garre K, Rasmussen K, Erenlund Jensen H (1990) Quality of life as outcome measure in mild hypertension (in Danish). Ugeskr Laeger 152:383–386

Derogatis LR, Lipman RS, Rickels K, Uhlenhuth EH, Covi L (1974) The Hopkins symptom checklist (HSCL). In: Pichot P (ed) Psychological measurement in psychopharmacology, Karger, Basel, pp 79–110

Eysenck HJ, Eysenck SBG (1976) Psychoticism as a dimension of personality. Hodder and Stonghton, London

Frank JD (1974) Persuasion and healing. Schocken, New York

Goldberg D (1972) The detection of psychiatric illness by questionnaire. Oxford University Press, Oxford

Griffin J (1986) Well-being. Its meaning, measurement and moral importance. Oxford, Clarendon

Guy W (ed) (1976) Early clinical drug evaluation program (ECDEV). Assessment manual. Department of Health, Education and Welfare, Rockwill, pp 218–222

Hamilton M (1960) A rating scale for depression. J Neurol Neurosurg Psychiatry 23:56–62

Holden JMC, Hsu W, Itil TM, Keskiner A (1971) Predictor patterns in the management of therapy-resistant schizophrenia. Dis Nerv Syst 32:260–268

Holmes TJ, Rahe RH (1967) The social readjustment rating scale. J Psychosom Res 11:213–218

Hunt SM, McKenna SP, McEwen J, Williams J, Papp E (1981) The Nottingham health profile: subjective health status and medical consultations. Soc Sci Med 15:221–229

Levine RRJ, Fogg L, Meltzer HY (1983) Assessment of negative and positive symptoms in schizophrenia. Schizophr Bull 9:368–375

Likert RA (1932) A technique for the measurement of attitudes. Arch Psychol 140:1–55

Lingjærde O, Ahlfors UG, Bech P, Dencker SJ, Elgen K (1987) The UKU side effect rating scale. Acta Psychiatr Scand 76[Suppl 326]:1–100

MacMillan AM (1957) The health opinion survey: technique for estimating prevalence of psychoneurotic and related types of disorder in communities. Psychol Rep 3:325–339

Miller GA (1956) The magical number of seven, plus or minus two. Psychol Rev 63:81–97

Overall JE (1979) Criteria for the selection of subjects for research in biological psychiatry. In: van Pragh HM, Lader MH, Rafaelsen OJ, Sachar EJ (eds) Handbook of biological psychiatry. Dekker, New York, pp 359–391

Parloff MB (1970) Assessing the effects of headshrinking and mind-expanding. Int J Group Psychother 1:14–24

Parloff MB, Kelman HC, Frank JD (1954) Comfort, effectiveness and self-awareness as criteria of improvement in psychotherapy. Am J Psychiatry 111:343–351

Stevens SS (1962) The surprising simplicity of sensory metrics. Am Psychol 17:29–39

Thurstone LL (1928) Attitudes can be measured. Am J Sociol 33:529–554

Veroff J, Fels S, Gurin G (1962) Dimensions of subjective adjustment. J Abnorm Soc Psychol 64:192–198

Wenger NK, Mattson ME, Furberg CD, Elinson J (1984) Assessment of quality of life in clinical trials of cardiovascular therapies. Am J Cardiol 54:908–913

# Ascertainment of Side Effects in Psychopharmacologic Clinical Trials*

J. Levine[1]

## 1 Background

Since the era of modern pharmacologic treatment of psychiatric disorders began in the mid-1950s, much progress has been made in techniques to assess the efficacy of proposed therapeutic agents. This has come about for a variety of reasons including the amendment to the U.S. Food, Drug, and Cosmetics Law in 1962 that requires proof of efficacy before marketing of prescription medications is permitted. Assessment or proof of safety prior to marketing had been a requirement for many years.

One might assume, therefore, that the methodology for assessing safety would be more highly developed and more satisfactory than that for assessing efficacy, but this is certainly not the case. In fact, a fully acceptable and operationally useful definition of safety probably has not yet been achieved. Again, there are multiple reasons for this, including both value issues and scientific-technical problems. Efforts of the pharmaceutical industry, the Food and Drug Administration (FDA), and the medical-scientific drug assessment community, over the 20 years following the enactment of the Harris Kefauver Amendment focussed heavily on assessing efficacy, while safety issues remained more in the background as a necessary but not sufficient condition for marketing.

In many ways, assessment of efficacy is a more straightforward technical issue. With the advent of the controlled clinical trial emphasizing random assignment of patients to treatment and techniques such as blinding to reduce bias and quantitative rating scales to improve accuracy of measurement of outcome, all that is needed for efficacy assessment is a good definition of the disorder to be treated and a representative sample of patients with the disorder. Clinical trials, and especially those studying treatment of psychiatric disorders, are designed primarily to assure adequate efficacy assessment (Peace 1987).

Safety assessment presents a host of other problems. In contrast to efficacy assessment, there is no sample of patients with the symptom or disorder, which can be used as an inclusion criterion for the trial. The symptom or side effect may

* Preparation of this chapter was partially supported by a Clinical Research Center Grant, MH40279, from the National Institute of Mental Health.

[1] Maryland Psychiatric Research Center, University of Maryland, Department of Psychiatry, P.O. Box 21247, Baltimore, MD 21228, USA

Methodology of the Evaluation of Psychotropic Drugs
Editors: O. Benkert, W. Maier, and K. Rickels
(Psychopharmacology Series 8)
© Springer-Verlag Berlin Heidelberg 1990

occur in any body system, whether physical or mental, and there must be a system to detect the wide band of side effects. In addition to the broad range problem, the frequency of occurrence of most side effects is quite low; thus the detection system must be very sensitive and not miss these rather infrequently occurring events. The power to detect a side effect is thus generally lower than the power to detect an efficacy effect in the usual clinical trial. Furthermore, since side effects tend to be individual symptoms rather than syndromes (profile of symptoms), the cause or etiology is much more difficult to attribute with certainty. The disorder under treatment or intercurrent illnesses frequently give rise to symptoms which can result in false positive or false negative conclusions about whether the symptom is a side effect (drug related) or not.

Given this range of problems, what conceptualization, technique, or methodologies may be employed to address these problems? First, the entire conundrum of safety assessment must be analytically dissected into a number of smaller, more manageable and addressable components. It is useful, for example, to separate the problem of detecting rare but serious side effects from detecting those that may be important, but less severe, and of more frequent occurrence. The latter are part of the pharmacologic profile of the drug and are more likely to be dose related. Over the past 10 years, a greater effort has been made in developing techniques to identify the former, i.e., rare but serious events. These techniques have focussed on postmarketing surveillance (because of the large number of patients receiving the drug) and on developing algorithms to establish whether the rare event can be causally attributed to the drug. Postmarketing surveillance can use intensive inpatient monitoring (Jick et al. 1970; Speiss-Kiefer et al. 1988), voluntary reporting (Faich 1986), and in-person or telephone interviewing techniques with patients in outpatient status (Fisher et al. 1987; Mellinger et al. 1988). Algorithms range from logical checklist approaches (Stephens 1985) to more formal probabalistic models (Jones and Herman 1986). Frequently the number of cases with the adverse event is very small (between one and five), while the number of patients receiving the drug is very large but the number is inexactly known.

In the regulatory area, at least in the United States, the FDA has a separate Office/Division receiving postmarketing surveillance data and analyzing this data for previously unidentified adverse drug reactions. Emphasis is therefore on the rare and serious side effects. Likewise, in the reviewing divisions (organized according to therapeutic classes), while some estimates of the rate of nonserious side effects are determined in reviewing a new drug application, the decision to market is usually based on the absence of serious side effects and evidence of efficacy.

From a scientific and clinical-medical perspective, the nonserious side effects are quite important. This is especially the case in the area of psychopharmacologic agents, where differences in the therapeutic efficacy of agents within a class (e.g., neuroleptics, antidepressants, or anxiolytics) are minimal or nonexistent while side effects are nontrivially different. Non-life-threatening side effects may be annoying enough for patients not to comply and cooperate in taking the prescribed medication, thus having a significant effect on efficacy. Therefore, information needs to be accumulated during premarketing clinical trials that will be sufficient for practitioners to prescribe and monitor drug therapy knowledgeably. From a scientific perspective, minor side effects (mild hypotension, slight fever) may signal the potential of major adverse drug reactions (severe orthostatic hypotension, serum sickness-like reactions) in rare cases when the drug is received by hundreds of thousands or millions of individuals. The accurate detection of nonserious side effects in the context of clinical trials will be the focus of the remainder of this chapter.

## 2 Ascertainment Issues

Surprisingly little literature is available providing empirical evidence on reliable and valid methods for collecting side effect data (Downing et al. 1970; Petrie and Levine 1978; Koeppen et al. 1989). A major methodological problem in this area is the lack of an external criterion by which to judge the accuracy of different ascertainment techniques. After reading reports of many clinical trials and protocols in psychopharmacology and discussing methods with sponsors and principal investigators, it is rather clear that the methods used both across trials and within trials are frequently unsystematic. Even without empirical data this leads to the conclusion that, because of this nonuniform approach, there must be greater variability in results reported (and hence less reliability) than if a systematic approach were used. Some of the areas which need to be systematized are presented below.

## 3 Voluntary Versus Elicited Inquiry and Total Versus Drug Related Reporting

The method by which a rater or examiner obtains information on whether an adverse health event (and hence a potential side effect) has occurred varies between pure voluntary reporting (depending entirely on a patient's spontaneous report) and use of a detailed checklist of events, for which each of the events is directly and explicitly inquired about from each patient (usually at repeated intervals). Again the point is made that, while there are advocates for each approach (and for the more reasonable middle ground between), at least the approach used in a given trial should be explicit and uniform. Those who believe in spontaneous reporting claim that serious events will clearly emerge (information) and not be overwhelmed by meaningless "noise" created when specific elicitation suggests events to patients. Those who believe in elicited inquiry feel that, without an elicitation, many events which could be drug related are not reported and an underestimate of unexpected events occurs. This question can be reformulated into an issue of specificity and sensitivity (Fletcher et al. 1982), which is usually reserved for accuracy of diagnostic tests and epidemiologic studies. In fact, the author has reanalyzed data provided by Markowitz et al. (1987) with results showing that specific inquiry has much greater sensitivity and only a slightly reduced specificity than a general inquiry procedure (Levine and Schooler 1986). Since this result was based on limited data from a single clinical trial, other data and studies are needed to see if this finding is generalizable to other drugs and patient samples.

The issue of total versus drug related reporting is as follows. In some clinical trials, if an adverse health event is reported by the patient (spontaneously or as a result of elicitation), the examiner is instructed to report (record) it only if it is suspected to be drug related (unless it is life-threatening, so severe that the drug must be stopped, the patient hospitalized, or contra-active medication used). This type of reporting is very likely to lead to under-reporting of unexpected and unanticipated adverse health events relative to those that are known or expected. Total event reporting (Skegg and Doll 1977) does not put a burden on the examiner to decide whether an event is drug related or not, but attempts to determine this by means of group, not individual patient data from the trial. Clearly, the author favors the latter approach.

## 4 Extent of Event Information

Once the decision has been made that an adverse health event has occurred, there is great diversity in what information about the event needs to be collected. To start with, should there be some standardized list of preferred event terms or should the examiner use the term he feels is most descriptive? Alternatively, should the patients own words be recorded verbatim? The author favors the first alternative. This is based on the proposition that when the data from multiple patients are tabulated, it is necessary to group the same or similar events, and problems of postcoding then occur. It is far better to have the examiner carefully ascertain from the patient the best description of the symptom (event) and then assign it a preferred term designation (code) rather than having someone who has never seen the patient try to make the determination. This assumes that the examiner will have a health science background (e.g., physician, nurse, pharmacist). Obviously, if no appropriate preferred term exists on the list, then the examiner uses best judgement and includes the patient's own words. To facilitate the use of a preferred term list, the terms should be organized separately by alphabetical order and by body system (e.g., gastrointestinal, cardiovascular, neurological). Providing a list of symptoms considered to be equivalent (synonyms) but not preferred is also very helpful.

While having the event named is the single most important piece of information, it is usually not sufficient by itself to interpret the importance of the event or to help in making an attribution of cause (e.g., drug related or not). In terms of importance, severity and reversibility (or lasting consequence) are crucial, along with the action taken by the clinician. There are several aspects of severity. Certain events, e.g., seizure, are considered to be of greater medical significance than, for example, dry mouth. However, ascertaining the severity within a given event is also important. This can be separated into severity of reported distress and severity based on interference with other physiological or behavioral activities (i.e., functional impairment). Separately, knowing whether the event is continuing, terminated, or has left sequelae is crucial for interpreting the importance of the event. Another behavioral measure of importance is the action taken by the clinician in response to the event, e.g., no action taken or patient dropped from the study.

To help in attributing cause, having the time of onset, duration, pattern (isolated, continuing), and other possible contributory factors (e.g., intercurrent illness) are essential. That is not to say that the occurrence of each event in each patient should be causally attributed by the investigator, but the totality of experience with the event in the trial is likely to be better understood when the above information is available. The primary method of testing for attribution to drug in the controlled clinical trial is, of course, by statistically testing between experimental and control groups for the frequency of the event.

Relating dosage or time on drug to occurrence of the event also can provide evidence of drug related causality (O'Neill 1988).

## 5 Specification of Time Period

Being explicit about the time frame to which the inquiry refers is another necessary systematization. Does the inquiry refer to the last week, to the period since the last inquiry, or solely to the present moment? The decision as to what time frame to use is an example of a protocol driven decision, that is, depending on the design of the trial and the questions being asked, the most appropriate time frame is selected and applied uniformly and explicitly during the trial. If the trial calls for a comparison between a predrug administration period and a time period while on drug, then the baseline period inquired about should be of equivalent duration to the on drug period. For example, if the trial is to test the efficacy and safety of a new antidepressant and patients are seen weekly to rate efficacy and safety, then the period inquired about at baseline should be 1 week. Frequency of occurrence of any given event, e.g., headache, is compared for each 1 week period in the trial on drug to the 1 week period (baseline) prior to onset of drug treatment. Cumulative frequency over the 6 week period can be compared with cumulative frequency of a concurrent comparison drug (standard) or placebo if one was included in the trial.

## 6 Conclusion

By providing uniformity in the above three discussed domains, the quality of the data collected for ascertainment of side effects will be vastly improved over what is now common practice. The variability of response in the data will be reduced and hence the ability to detect side effects enhanced. A rating device which incorporates this degree of standardization for side effect assessment is the SAFTEE (Systematic Assessment For Treatment Emergent Events) (Levine and Schooler 1986). While this is not the only format or content of an instrument which could incorporate the principles of standardization presented above, it represents a concrete example, which can be modified or built upon much as rating scales for efficacy assessment have been developed and diversified over time.

## References

Downing RW, Rickels K, Meyers F (1970) Side reactions in neurotics: a comparison of two methods of assessment. J Clin Pharmacol 10:289–297

Faich GA (1986) Adverse drug reaction monitoring. N Engl J Med 314:1589–1592

Fisher S, Bryant SG, Kluge RM (1987) Detecting adverse drug reactions in post marketing surveillance: interview-validity. Drug Inform J 21:173–183

Fletcher RH, Fletcher SW, Wagner EH (1982) Clinical epidemiology – the essentials. Williams and Wilkins, Baltimore

Jick H, Miettinen OS, Shapiro S et al. (1970) Comprehensive drug surveillance. J Am Med Assoc 215:1455–1460

Jones JK, Herman RL (1986) The future of adverse drug reaction diagnosis: computers, clinical judgement and the logic of uncertainty. Drug Inform J 20/4:445–535

Koeppen K, Mohr R, Streichenwein SM (1989) Assessment of adverse drug events during the clinical investigation of a new drug. Pharmacopsychiatry 22:93–98

Levine J, Schooler NR (1986) SAFTEE: a technique for the systematic assessment of side effects in clinical trials. Psychopharmacol Bull 22:343–381

Markowitz JS, Rabkin JG, Stewart J, Tricamo E, McGrath PJ, Harrison W, Ocepek-Welikson K, Quitkin FM (1987) Validity assessment of SAFTEE: a preliminary report. Psychopharmacol Bull 23:102–105

Mellinger GD, Balter MB, Abramowitz S, Schaffer CB, Bernstein LR (1988) Survey method for post marketing drug surveillance. J Clin Psychopharmacol 8:168–176

O'Neill RT (1988) Assessment of Safety. In: Peace KE (ed) Biopharmaceutical statistics for drug development. Dekker, New York

Peace KE (1987) Design, monitoring and analysis issues relative to adverse events. Drug Inform J 21:21–28

Petrie WM, Levine J (1978) The assessment of adverse reactions in clinical trials. Int Pharmacopsychiatry 13:209–216

Skegg D, Doll R (1977) The case for recording events in clinical trials. Br Med J 2:1523–1524

Speiss-Kiefer C, Grohmann R, Schmidt LG, Ruther E (1988) Six years of drug surveillance in psychiatric inpatients. Pharm Med 3:341–348

Stephens MDP (1985) The detection of new adverse drug reactions. Macmillan, London

# Selection Criteria for Drug Trials

# Diagnoses as Selection Criteria in Drug Trials

R. Buller and W. Maier[1]

## 1 Introduction

Drug trials are needed to establish the efficacy and safety of psychopharmacological agents in clearly defined indications. When the goal of treatment is more complex than removal of an isolated symptom ("difficulty in falling asleep" or "pain") the syndrome or clinical entity to be treated is most easily classified by way of a diagnostic label (like "depression," "schizophrenia," or "panic disorder"). Dimensional models have many advantages: they often fit the data better and provide a conceptual framework for a continuum in the behavior from normal to abnormal. However, they have never reached the popularity of typological models (Strauss 1973, 1975, 1986) which reflect more the medical thinking in the form of categories (like health versus illness). Clinical practice in psychiatry also favors the use of diagnostic categories for indication and selection of patients for treatment.

This paper discusses the problems associated with our present systems of classification for schizophrenia, mood disorders, and anxiety disorders, and their role in psychopharmacology. Other important conditions (like organic brain syndromes, dementia personality disorders, or sexual dysfunction) were not included for reasons of space.

## 2 Diagnostic Classification in Psychiatry

### 2.1 Validity

For most psychiatric disorders a specific etiology is unknown. Since there are no objective ways like biological tests or imaging techniques to prove structural lesions or functional abnormalities in order to determine the presence of disease, phenomenology is the basis of classification and clinical signs and symptoms are condensed into a diagnosis. Since symptoms are nonspecific, evidence is needed to support the hypothesis that a combination of symptoms or a syndrome is in fact a valid clinical entity.

[1] Psychiatrische Klinik der Universität Mainz, Untere Zahlbacher Str. 8, 6500 Mainz, FRG

Methodology of the Evaluation of Psychotropic Drugs
Editors: O. Benkert, W. Maier, and K. Rickels
(Psychopharmacology Series 8)
© Springer-Verlag Berlin Heidelberg 1990

**Table 1.** Validation criteria for psychiatric diagnosis (Robins and Guze 1970)

| | |
|---|---|
| 1. Clinical description | (content validity) |
| 2. Laboratory studies | (concurrent validity) |
| 3. Delimitation from other disorders | (construct validity) |
| 4. Follow-up study | (predictive validity) |
| 5. Family study | (criterion-related validity) |

Validity describes the extent to which categories reflect clinical reality. A stepwise process of validation was proposed by Robins and Guze (1970; see Table 1). In their concept "response to treatment" does not constitute a major criterion of validity by itself but may be subsumed as one aspect of outcome to be determined during follow-up.

For the classical diagnostic entities a validation by treatment outcome data is of limited value because most diagnostic categories in psychiatry originate before the development of the modern psychopharmacological agents and antipsychotics (neuroleptics), antidepressants (tricyclics, MAO inhibitors), and anxiolytics (tranquilizers, benzodiazepines) have been synthesized, without knowledge of their potential properties in psychiatric disorders.

Many drugs now used in psychiatry are capable of inducing various different effects. All have limited specificity in conditions defined by classical diagnoses. Independently of the specific formulation of the diagnostic criteria, the rate of nonresponders in major psychiatric categories appears to average around 30%. Since response and failure to respond to treatment seem to be differing also from time to time in the same patient (Cole 1988) they are probably not trait markers.

Because of these difficulties the value of a diagnosis for choice of a pharmacological treatment may be limited and is therefore a subject of debate. However, in a newly developed "functional classification" that is proposed by Benkert (this volume) treatment response serves as an important axis. In his approach the author calls for a classification which is specifically tailored for drug evaluation and is not only relying on psychopathology but considers other axes and variables like biological markers and physiological parameters. This could eventually lead to a renunciation of the principle of psychopathologically defined nosological entities at least in psychopharmacology if not in biological psychiatry.

## 2.2 Reliability

Specificity of drug action will also be missed when groups of psychiatric patients in whom efficacy of treatment is tested are heterogeneous because the criteria for definition of the illness are too ambiguous and unreliable. As a consequence, more reliable diagnostic categories have been called for (Spitzer et al. 1975, 1978) and developed in recent years. Systems like the Feighner Criteria (Feighner et al. 1972) and the Research Diagnostic Criteria (RDC) by Spitzer and coworkers

(1970) give operationalized definitions for a limited number of more frequently appearing psychiatric disorders.

Two clinical systems attempt to completely cover psychiatry: the *International Classification of Diseases, 9th Revision* (ICD-9) of the World Health Organization (WHO 1978) and the *Diagnostic and Statistical Manual of Mental Disorders, Third Edition, DSM-III* (American Psychiatric Association 1980) and its latest revision the DSM-III-R (American Psychiatric Association 1987). For both systems revisions are scheduled to appear after 1992 (ICD-10, DSM-IV) with the intent of developing specific research criteria in the ICD-10.

At present, the most widely recommended systems of classification in drug trials are the DSM-III and the DSM-III-R because both use operationalized criteria. They also attempt to combine categorical and dimensional approaches by introducing a multiaxial system, that allows for multiple diagnoses in which symptomatology and etiology are separated. Assessment is made on separate axes for psychopathological syndromes, personality disorders, physical diseases, severity of psychosocial stressors, and global functioning, but there is no separate axis to code the course of the disorder. For the DSM-III agreement was tested in field trials and proved to be sufficient for major diagnostic groups with kappa coefficients of 0.69 for affective disorders, of 0.81 for schizophrenia, and of 0.63 for anxiety disorders (American Psychiatric Association 1980).

Reliability is increased by structured clinical interviews (Maier et al. 1988; Buller et al. 1988) which help to standardize the procedure of gathering the information necessary to make a diagnostic decision concerning the algorithms stated in the classification.

Such instruments like the Present State Examination PSE (Wing et al. 1974), the Schedule for Affective Disorders and Schizophrenia SADS (Endicott and Spitzer 1978), the Diagnostic Interview Schedule DIS (Robins et al. 1981), the Structured Clinical Interview for DSM-III SCID (Spitzer and Williams 1983), the Composite International Diagnostic Interview CIDI (Robins et al. 1985), and the Polydiagnostic Interview PODI (Philipp and Maier, 1986) are widely used in diagnostic assessment for specific classification systems. The Schedules for Clinical Assessment in Neuropsychiatry SCAN (Wing 1988) is an interview based on the PSE, which allows for polydiagnostic assessment (see Table 2).

The existence of different diagnostic systems suggests that none is completely satisfactory with respect to validity and reliability. Still, there is a basic consensus that a "state-of-the-art" is needed for making a clinical diagnosis and for treatment which has to consider our present concepts and should reflect on current developments in empirical research.

## 3 Diagnostic Categories in Psychopharmacology

When the efficacy of a compound is tested and compared with a reference drug or placebo, the respective groups of the sample have to be similar and homogeneous in their basic characteristics. The clinical information on the condition is in part contained in the diagnosis. Other variables like age, gender,

**Table 2.** Classification systems and diagnostic interviews for schizophrenia, depression, and anxiety disorders

| System | Operational criteria | Structured diagnostic interview |
|---|---|---|
| ICD-9 | No | none, (PSE[a]) |
| CATEGO | Yes | PSE, CIDI |
| Feighner criteria | Yes | PODI, DIS, CIDI |
| RDC | Yes | DIS, SADS, PODI, CIDI, SCAN[c] |
| DSM-III | Yes | SCID, SADS, PODI, (DIS[a]) |
| DSM-III-R | Yes | PODI, (SCID[b], SADS[c]) |
| DSM-IV[d] | Yes | [c] |
| ICD-10[d] | Yes | SCAN[c], CIDI |

[a] Covers only part of the criteria.
[b] Revision due shortly.
[c] In preparation, not available.
[d] In preparation, scheduled to appear 1992, 1993.

prior psychiatric history, length of previous treatment, nature and number of prior episodes, level of functioning, duration of current episode, severity of illness, and inpatient or outpatient status need to be ascertained, as well.

In diagnostic systems (like DSM-III) that use a hierarchy to explain the relationship between symptoms and individual diagnostic categories, in cases with a "higher" disorder, like organic mental disorder, a diagnosis of schizophrenia or a co-existing affective or anxiety syndrome is not made even when the inclusion criteria for these disorders are met since the symptoms are judged to be caused by an organic mental disorder. In the DSM-III the hierarchical order of the syndromes and disorders is stated in the form of exclusion criteria. Organic brain syndromes are placed on the highest level in all circumstances and have to be ruled out before a diagnosis of another disorder (like schizophrenia or depression) can be made. The diagnosis of schizophrenia excludes a diagnosis of major depression and vice versa. In cases with both psychotic and affective symptomatology (but with no indication for an organic brain syndrome) a decision has to be made whether the psychotic symptoms are secondary or brief with respect to the full affective syndrome (leading, e.g., to a diagnosis of major depression with psychotic features) or whether the affective symptomatology is superimposed on schizophrenia (leading to a diagnosis of schizophrenia, possibly with atypical depression). Only when the clinician is unable to make a differential diagnosis between schizophrenia and affective disorder is the diagnosis of schizoaffective disorder given (however, there are no explicit criteria in the DSM-III for this condition). There is another hierarchy between the affective disorders and the anxiety disorders: a specific anxiety disorder is only diagnosed when the symptoms are not due to depression (or another disorder like schizophrenia).

Drug trials which aim at very narrowly defined groups may use diagnoses as additional criteria for exclusion. An example can be taken from the Cross-National Collaborative Panic Study (1989) in which the following psychiatric conditions (besides some somatic illnesses) led to exclusion of the patient from the trial: lifetime history of epilepsy, psychotic disorder, drug-induced psychosis, dementia, bipolar disorder, melancholic or psychotic depression, primary depression, cyclothymic disorder, alcoholism, drug abuse, and obsessive-compulsive disorder.

At the present time, diagnoses in psychopharmacological research should serve the following purposes:

1. To identify homogeneous groups concerning the illness in question (criteria for inclusion and exclusion).
2. To predict response to treatment and failure to respond to placebo or spontaneously.
3. To communicate findings within the scientific community and to allow for generalization of the results.
4. To help formulate concepts and to develop theories that fit the data.

Besides being valid and reliable, the wording of the criteria used in the diagnosis has to be meaningful, adaptable, and translatable so that they can be used internationally. They should also be compatible with measures of severity and change (like rating scales) that are used to quantify the effect of the treatment.

## 4 Drug Trials in Specific Psychiatric Disorders

For some major psychiatric disorders problems and requirements concerning the use of diagnostic categories in relation to drug trials will be discussed in more detail.

### 4.1 Schizophrenia

Pharmacotherapy in schizophrenia is not limited to the treatment of acute states of the illness but also has to deal with maintenance treatment and the prevention of relapse. Diagnostic criteria should help with the search for predictors of response, nonresponse, and relapse, so that therapists can identify patients in need of prolonged treatment.

Even in the first descriptions of schizophrenia by Kraepelin and Bleuler, the syndrome was conceptualized as a group of conditions which had in common an early onset and a chronic, deteriorating course. Competing definitions have been proposed, since then, with considerable overlap among them. Differences concerning symptomatology, age of onset, duration, and hierarchical exclusion criteria (e.g., mood disorders) result in various degrees of restrictiveness in the different systems (see Table 3).

Depending on the system used for diagnosis, the mode of recruitment of patients for drug trials may differ considerably. Acute cases which would already

**Table 3.** Classification systems for diagnosis of schizophrenia

| System | Minimal duration of symptoms | Age of onset (years) | Restrictiveness |
|---|---|---|---|
| ICD-9 | – | – | Moderate |
| Feighner criteria | 6 Months | Before 40 | Narrow |
| RDC | 2 Weeks | – | Narrow |
| DSM-III | 6 Months | Before 45 | Narrow |
| DSM-III-R | 6 Months | Before 45[a] | Narrow |
| DSM-IV[b] | ? | ? | ? |
| ICD-10[b] | ? | ? | ? |

[a] Otherwise specify "late onset".
[b] In preparation, scheduled to appear 1992, 1993.

be diagnosed as schizophrenia by ICD-9 can be recruited as inpatients in a university hospital or even in outpatient departments. Studies which use DSM-III criteria call for more chronic cases with a longer prior course or previous episodes and may have to be carried out in facilities like state mental hospitals (unless patients with the diagnosis of schizophreniform disorder are also included). The DSM-III and the DSM-III-R form a compromise in emphasizing cross-sectional features (delusions, hallucinations, and thought disorder). However, both take into consideration that the course of the disorder is often chronic: to qualify, the patient has to have symptoms for at least 6 months. However, in DSM-III-R, criteria have undergone revision already, leading to criticism like that by Fenton et al. (1988) who reported that patients who met DSM-III criteria but were excluded from the diagnosis of schizophrenia by DSM-III-R were not different with respect to demographic, premorbid, and long-term outcome variables.

Within any known system for classification of schizophrenia subtypes have been proposed to explain the variance in symptoms, course, outcome, and treatment response (see Table 4).

So far, there is no strong predictive ability for short-term treatment response to neuroleptics for any of the classical subtypes of schizophrenia (paranoid, disorganized/hebephrenic, or catatonic). For patients with residual schizophrenia, separate trials need to be conducted for test of efficacy.

In order to explore reasons for nonresponse to neuroleptic treatment, Andreasen and Olsen (1982) defined two different types of schizophrenia. They are characterized by either positive symptoms (like hallucinations or delusions) which are supposed to respond to neuroleptics or negative, nonresponsive symptoms (like lack of volition). The authors postulate that the two types are associated with either specific biochemical changes in receptors or structural changes in brain tissue. However, Moscarelli et al. (1987) report on a large portion (75%) of their sample with mixed features of positive and negative symptoms. These data are in line with a concept proposed by Crow (1980) who does not

**Table 4.** Diagnostic subgroups (subtypes) in schizophrenia

| Subtype | System(s) |
|---|---|
| Simple schizophrenia | ICD-9 |
| Disorganized schizophrenia | DSM-III, DSM-III-R |
| Catatonic schizophrenia | DSM-III, DSM-III-R, RDC, ICD-9 |
| Paranoid schizophrenia | DSM-III, DSM-III-R, RDC, ICD-9 |
| Undifferentiated schizophrenia | DSM-III, DSM-III-R, RDC, ICD-9 |
| Residual schizophrenia | DSM-III, DSM-III-R, RDC, ICD-9 |
| Acute schizophrenic episode | RDC, ICD-9 |
| Subchronic, chronic schizophrenia with/without acute exacerbation | RDC, DSM-III, DSM-III-R |
| In remission | DSM-III, DSM-III-R |
| Positive/negative schizophrenia | Andreasen and Olsen (1982) |
| Type I/Type II schizophrenia | Crow (1980) |
| Conditions possibly related to schizophrenic disorders | |
| Latent schizophrenia | ICD-9 |
| Atypical | ICD-9 |
| Schizophreniform disorder | DSM-III, DSM-III-R |
| Schizoaffective psychosis | RDC, DSM-III-R, ICD-9 |
| Borderline personality disorder | DSM-III, DSM-III-R |
| Schizoid personality disorder | DSM-III, DSM-III-R |
| Schizotypal personality disorder | DSM-III, DSM-III-R |

regard "type I (positive)" and "type II (negative symptoms) schizophrenia" as mutually exclusive types of illness but as an independent dimensions that reflect different underlying disease processes. Although these new manners of subdivision seem to have some predictive validity for choice of treatment, there are still problems with the boundaries of these subtypes. It is not clear whether some of the features (like inappropriate affect) should be included with negative or positive symptoms. In addition, Liddle (1987) when questioning the positive-negative dichotomy found evidence for the existence of a third subtype characterized by poverty of speech and retardation.

For drug trials it is necessary to stratify the samples with respect to the presence or absence or severity of negative symptoms.

The validity of certain ill-defined conditions like latent or atypical schizophrenia (ICD-9) and their relation to the classic syndrome is not established, yet. It should be stated clearly when patients with these syndromes are included in efficacy studies. Although neuroleptics play an important role in the treatment of schizophreniform or schizoaffective disorder and in borderline personality disorder and schizotypal personality disorder, as well, so far the relation between any of these conditions and schizophrenia is not well understood. Research on any of these should be carried out separately in "pure" subsamples using well-defined diagnostic criteria (see Table 4).

Variability in prognosis that is not explained by diagnostic subtype might be reduced further by taking into account duration (chronicity) and severity of the disorder (Cloninger et al. 1985). In the future, a biological approach to delimit the diversity of the conditions that fall into the group of schizophrenias may involve the use of techniques like receptor studies, molecular genetics, family studies, and advanced imaging techniques to define more homogeneous subtypes or syndromal entities (DeLisi et al. 1986).

In the systematic search for efficacious therapeutic alternatives a clear definition for treatment-resistant schizophrenia is necessary. The present therapeutic strategies in these patients involve use of ECT and higher dosage of neuroleptics which also carries a greater risk of side effects. Reasons for altered and insufficient response to treatment may be due to patient characteristics that can be subsumed under a diagnostic label (e.g., specific symptomatology, course, chronicity). In addition, lack of response may be due to structural changes like brain atrophy that is seen in some patients. Other reasons for inefficacy of drugs may be related to pharmacological variables like insufficient dose, low plasma concentration, or variation in receptor sensitivity, although no clear correlations between dose and response or plasma level and response have been proven so far (Csernansky et al. 1985). The duration of the current episode of schizophrenia might be a predictor of response to treatment itself and should be used as a stratification variable in a drug trial. The general consensus across the overwhelming majority of classification schedules for schizophrenia (like DSM-III, DSM-III-R, RDC, ICD-10, Feighner Criteria) is that the Schneiderian first rank symptoms are the crucial diagnostic criteria. Consequently, the main selection criterion should be the cross-sectional symptomatology defined by Schneiderian "First Rank Symptoms" using DSM-III-R, RDC, or ICD-10. Instead of using an arbitrary criterion of minimum duration (1 month or even 6 months) samples should be stratified for this variable in pharmacological trials.

## 4.2 Mood Disorders

Drug trials in patients with mood disorders test the efficacy in (a) acute depressive or manic symptomatology for (b) maintenance treatment during remission of an acute episode and (c) prevention of relapse in patients with recurrent course.

For the classification of mood disorders a variety of systems like the Feighner Criteria, RDC, and the DSM-III/DSM-III-R list operational criteria for various depressive syndromes and subtypes. Although there is only partial validity for these subtypes, operational systems are preferred in research settings because their diagnostic categories are more reliable than those contained in the ICD-9. Higher reliability results from the use of structured diagnostic interviews (see Table 2).

With respect to mania there seems to be no major controversy except concerning the validity of a subtype with mood-incongruent psychotic features.

It is therefore recommended to study this subgroup of patients separately or to control for mood-incongruent features in drug trials.

Diagnoses for depressive syndromes consist of inclusion criteria (related to type of symptoms, duration, and severity) and exclusion criteria, which reflect hierarchical rules in the classification system. For example, psychotic symptoms rule out a diagnosis of dysthymia or cyclothymia according to DSM-III; organic brain syndrome or schizophrenia exclude patients from the diagnosis of major depression. Subtypes which have been defined to reduce the heterogeneity of broad categories like major depression (see Table 5) are not always mutually exclusive (Prusoff et al. 1980).

Further research on subtypes is warranted because there appear to be clinically relevant differences in response to treatment:

1. Clinical aspects and the course of the illness with both manic and depressive episodes led to the distinction between unipolar and bipolar depression. In bipolar disorder acute episodes of mania respond to lithium salts. The same compounds are used for prophylactic treatment so that further episodes of illness can be prevented in up to 70% of the treated patients. However, there is a search for even more homogeneous subtypes (Cassano et al. 1988) for both bipolar (bipolar I, II, and III) and unipolar disorder (unipolar recurrent, unipolar single episode). At present, no evidence has been found for a different drug response to antidepressant for treatment of an acute depressive episode in unipolar and bipolar disorder.
2. Although the concept of endogenous depression (ICD-9) has been incorporated into the DSM-III, DSM-III-R, and RDC ("melancholic" or "endogenous" subtype) there is a continuing debate about the validity of this condition. A finding reported by Maier et al. (1988a) supports the validity of the concept. In their study the endogenous subgroup had an unfavorable course during the drug-free period in their study. Using various definitions of endogenous depression within a polydiagnostic approach, endogenomorphic features including diurnal variations and personality features were predictive for response to tricyclics (Maier et al. in press; Philipp and Maier 1988).
3. Patients with a delusional (psychotic) depression respond poorly to tricyclics alone, or may need longer time until response occurs (Howarth and Grace 1985) and often improve with additional medication with neuroleptics.
4. For situational depression a response to treatment with either interpersonal psychotherapy (IPT) or amitriptyline alone is reported, however response was even better for the combination of both, whereas patients with endogenous depression responded to amitriptyline alone, to a combination of amitriptyline with IPT but not to IPT alone (Prusoff et al. 1980). These findings need further replication.
5. Seasonal affective disorder is postulated to constitute a subtype of recurrent depression responsive to a "non-drug therapy" with light (Rosenthal et al. 1984).
6. Several studies report a more pronounced or at least faster response to tricyclics in primary than in secondary depression (Davidson and Pelton 1986; Maier et al., in press).

**Table 5.** Diagnostic subgroups in mood disorders

| Diagnosis/Subtype | Classification system |
|---|---|
| Major depressive episode/major depressive disorder | DSM-III, DSM-III-R, RDC, |
| With/without melancholia, endogenous features | DSM-III, DSM-III-R, RDC |
| With/without psychotic features | DSM-III, DSM-III-R, RDC |
| (Specify mood-congruent/-incongruent) | DSM-III, DSM-III-R |
| Primary/secondary depression | Feighner Criteria, RDC |
| Single episode | DSM-III, DSM-III-R |
| Recurrent unipolar | RDC, DSM-III, DSM-III-R |
| Inactivated | RDC |
| Agitated | RDC |
| Retarded | RDC |
| Situational | RDC |
| Simple | RDC |
| Seasonal pattern | DSM-III-R |
| Manic-depressive psychosis, depressed type (endogenous depression, involutional melancholia, monopolar depression, psychotic depression) | ICD-9 |
| Dysthymia | DSM-III, DSM-III-R |
| Primary/secondary | DSM-III-R |
| Early/late onset | DSM-III-R |
| Seasonal pattern | DSM-III-R |
| Depressive neurosis | ICD-9 |
| Minor depressive disorder | RDC |
| Other specific depressive disorders | |
| Characterological depression | Akiskal |
| Atypical depression | Quitkin et al. |
| Hysteroid dysphoria | Klein |
| Late luteal phase dysphoric disorder | DSM-III-R |
| Adjustment disorder with depressed mood | DSM-III, DSM-III-R |
| Brief depressive reaction | ICD-9 |
| Prolonged depressive reaction | ICD-9 |
| Bipolar disorders | |
| Manic episode (bipolar I) | DSM-III, DSM-III-R, RDC, Feighner |
| Manic-depressive psychosis, circular type but currently depressed (bipolar disorder, now depressed) | ICD-9 |
| Hypomanic syndrome (bipolar II) | RDC |
| Cyclothymia | DSM-III, DSM-III-R |

7. Subjects with atypical depression and with hysteroid dysphoria seem to be preferentially responsive to monoamine oxidase inhibitors (Liebowitz et al. 1988). An operational definition for atypical depression is not contained in the major classification systems but given by Quitkin et al. (1988). For the diagnosis the patient had to meet RDC criteria for minor or major depression. Their mood

had to be reactive mood and at least one out of four associated symptoms (hyperphagia, hypersomnolence, leaden feeling, and sensitivity to rejection) were required. However, there are competing concepts of the syndrome: (a) depression with associated panic, (b) depression secondary to a diagnosis of an anxiety disorder, and (c) depression with reversed vegetative signs. Whether the superiority of response to MAO inhibitors is related to the presence of panic attacks or to hysteroid dysphoric features or is different in female patients (Davidson and Pelton 1986) is still an open question.

But even when samples consist of apparently homogeneous subgroups (like nondelusional, unipolar melancholic inpatients, who have been depressed for less than 1 year) treatment response to adequate doses of tricyclics is still limited and found in approximately 80% of the patients. At present, prediction of a positive treatment response is not possible when predictors are only based on demographic data or clinical symptomatology (Roose et al. 1986; Joyce and Paykel 1989) with the possible exclusion of duration and personality features.

It has been stressed that although antidepressant medication can control the overt symptomatology there may be no immediate cure of the episode and prolonged treatment even after disappearance of mild symptoms may be necessary for some months (Prien and Kupfer 1986) in order to prevent relapse. This relates to the questions of how to measure outcome and how to determine improvement and remission (see Maier, this volume). Whereas improvement is often measured by way of change on ratings for severity, there is only limited consensus on the criteria for remission: patients may have to be "essentially free" of depressive symptoms. Alternatively, they may not meet the full criteria for the disorder any more without specifying the duration of this state (DSM-III). In the DSM-III-R there is a distinction between "partial remission" and "full remission" where the patient is without significant signs or symptoms for the past 6 months.

The overlap that is found between major depressive episode and chronic minor depression (dysthymia) is addressed by the term "double depression." Since hierarchical rules in classification have been dropped in the DSM-III-R for most disorders which are not due to organic diseases, comorbidity between alcohol abuse, anxiety disorders, and depressive disorders is expressed by dual diagnoses. With this more elaborate description of patients it is expected to illustrate and control variability in samples.

Dual diagnoses are also appropriate when the clinical presentation of a depressive disorder seems to be colored by personality variables or a personality disorder, which – besides duration of the episode – is the single consistent predictor for unfavorable response to tricyclics (Parker et al. 1988; Joyce and Paykel 1989). For long-standing problems due to affective symptomatology some authors have proposed categories like "affective personality disorder" and "cyclothymic temperamental disorders" (Akiskal et al. 1979) to reflect a lifelong pattern of affective symptomatology.

The former ICD-9 category of "neurotic depression" or "depressive neurosis" is now labeled "dysthymia." In the DSM-III the concept of dysthymic disorder includes chronic (persistent or intermittent) depressive symptoms for 2 years, subsyndromal intensity, not meeting full criteria for major depression, absence of psychotic features, and absence of hypomanic or manic mood swings (which would lead to a diagnosis of bipolar disorder or cyclothymic disorder). In spite of these seemingly specific criteria there is only limited data on the natural course and treatment response in this condition.

For other types of chronic (low grade) depression Akiskal (1983) has proposed a subclassification that separates (a) primary (late onset) depression with residual chronicity, (b) variable onset chronic secondary depression, and (c) early onset characterological depression with or without response to thymoleptic medication (subaffective dysthymic disorders vs character-spectrum disorders).

Formerly, new antidepressants were mainly tested in endogenous depression because other subtypes were believed not to respond to pharmacotherapy. As discussed, there is no major clinical evidence for this rationale. Therefore, major depressive episode defined by DSM-III is the main selection criterion for acute antidepressant drug trials in the majority of studies. An additional criterion for the baseline severity may be reasonable because of a finding reported by Paykel (1988) that efficacy of antidepressants below an initial HAMD score of 13 is questionable. However, replication of this study is needed. Major depression with psychotic features should be excluded in samples intended for the investigation of efficacy of a new antidepressant because of the overwhelming evidence for the relative inefficacy of monotherapy with antidepressants. Separate drug trials should be conducted for this condition.

Centers that carry out psychopharmacological research are often not the first facility that a patient will contact. This may lead to a high prevalence of patients with a chronic course and previous nonresponse to antidepressants. Drug trials should attempt to exclude patient groups with episodes longer than 3 months.

### 4.3 Anxiety Disorders

During recent years research into anxiety disorders has concentrated on the syndrome of panic disorder. Advances in this area are sometimes viewed as paradigmatic for the success of an empirical approach in search of drug responsive subgroups (Murphy et al. 1978). Characteristics of patients that remit with a certain medication have undergone systematic investigation in order to define specific (drug-responsive subtypes) among more global, mixed, or ill-defined conditions. In anxiety research this development started from the finding that the frequency of panic attacks could be reduced with continuous imipramine treatment and led to a "pharmacological dissection" (Klein et al. 1987) of the classical entity of "anxiety neurosis" into panic disorder (responsive to tricyclics but not to benzodiazepines) and generalized anxiety disorder (responsive to benzodiazepines but not to tricyclics). The use of operationalized diagnostic criteria and structured diagnostic interviews (see Table 2) that were translated into several different languages led to international research activities such as the projects on the safety and efficacy of alprazolam and imipramine versus placebo (Cross-National Collaborative Panic Study Second Phase Investigators, to be published).

Although there are different lines of evidence for the validity of panic disorder like experiments with lactate provocation and data from family studies (Fyer 1987) the question of the boundaries of the syndrome remains unsolved. There is a significant overlap and comorbidity with chronic (generalized) anxiety, agoraphobia, social phobia, and depression and substance abuse. Not only is there a distinction between different types of anxiety in various "distinct" anxiety disorders but also in the "single" condition of panic disorder where a line is drawn between panic attacks (specifically responsive to imipramine according to Klein et al.), anticipatory anxiety (nonresponsive to imipramine), phobic fears, and avoidance. The uncertainty about the validity of a separate diagnostic entity of panic disorder is also reflected in the rapid succession of continuously modified sets of diagnostic criteria (RDC, DSM-III, DSM-III-R, ICD-10). Recently, there is increasing evidence that the classification of the anxiety disorders possesses only limited prognostic validity concerning choice of drug and that there is merely limited specificity for the effectiveness of both groups of drug. Imipramine has been found to work well in generalized anxiety. Benzodiazepines like alprazolam, clonazepam, lorazepam, and possibly high doses of diazepam, as well, are now thought to prevent panic attacks (Noyes 1987; Holmberg 1987).

Drug response in other anxiety disorders like social phobia, obsessive-compulsive disorder, and posttraumatic stress disorder is less well understood and calls for increased research efforts. However, operational diagnostic criteria and structured interviews to ascertain the diagnosis are already available and mentioned in Table 2. In addition, there are interviews like the ADIS (DiNardo et al. 1985) specifically developed for anxiety research.

As long as it remains unclear whether various types of anxiety like panic disorder, generalized anxiety disorder, agoraphobia etc. differ in their drug response, pharmacological trials should either be conducted separately for each category or at least be balanced for the distinct disorders. Because there is a high amount of overlap between anxiety disorders and major depression which might induce a different response to drugs (especially in cases with primary major depression) drug trials for treatment of anxiety should exclude patients with primary major depression or should at least use this condition for stratification.

## 5 Conclusion

The development of more specific drug treatments and identification of predictors for drug-response will be a major goal for the immediate future. At present, the use of *clinical diagnoses* as selection criteria in trials on efficacy is still a common practice and a necessity in order to transfer new findings into routine application. However, in the future this practice may be overcome by "functional classifications" proposed by Benkert (this volume) that are tailored to directly identify (drug) treatment-responsive conditions. Until then, clinical criteria should stem from an official classification system. They should be broad enough, valid, and simple to use. Presence or absence of symptoms is best determined by experts using structured clinical instruments with sufficient reliability.

For more specialized biological investigations, narrow and strict *research criteria* may be necessary. However, they ought to be part of the broader clinical categories and the relation between these sets of criteria has to be formulated. The DSM-III and its revision DSM-III-R have been a start. For special research purposes criteria can be modified and still remain explicit (by changing the number of symptoms necessary, duration, or exclusion criteria). Possibly, the tenth revision of the International Classification of Diseases (ICD-10) will be another step in this direction (Cooper 1988).

In studies carried out in research settings, better use of data from empirical investigations can be achieved, when the description of patients is based on assessments by means of *polydiagnostic structured instruments* in ways that allow for assignment of multiple diagnoses from competing classification schemes. This procedure would permit to test the relevance of revised criteria and diagnostic algorithms by exact recording of presence, severity, and duration of relevant symptoms without loss of information due to arbitrary cut-offs and premature instructions to skip to different areas of the symptomatology. Shorter and less comprehensive versions could be prepared for clinical practice that use the same structure but need less time for completion.

The search for better classification systems based on empirical data will be – by its very nature – open to change, when new relevant findings are seen. In the future, modifications in classification will have to consider findings from psychopharmacological research. Possibly this will take the form of an additional axis for response to prior treatment.

## References

Akiskal HS (1983) Dysthymic disorder: psychopathology of proposed chronic depressive subtypes. Am J Psychiatry 140:11–20

Akiskal HS, Khani MK, Scott-Strauss A (1979) Cyclothymic temperamental disorders. Psychiatr Clin of North Am 3:527–554

American Psychiatric Association (1980) Diagnostic and statistical manual of mental disorders, third edition (DSM-III). American Psychiatric Association, Washington, DC

American Psychiatric Association (1987) Diagnostic and statistical manual of mental disorders, third edition, revised (DSM-III-R). American Psychiatric Association, Washington, DC

Andreasen NC, Olsen S (1982) Negative vs positive schizophrenia: definition and validation. Arch Gen Psychiatry 39:789–794

Buller R, Maier W, Philipp M (1988) Reliability of DSM-III anxiety disorders – check-list versus structured interview. Pharmacopsychiatry 6:422–423

Cassano GB, Musetti L, Perugi G, Soriani A, Mignani V, McNair DM, Akiskal HS (1988) A proposed new approach to the clinical subclassification of depressive illness. Pharmacopsychiatry 21:19–23

Cloninger RC, Martin RL, Guze SB, Clayton PJ (1985) Diagnosis and prognosis in schizophrenia. Arch Gen Psychiatry 42:15–25

Cole JO (1988) Where are those new antidepressants we were promised? Arch Gen Psychiatry 45:193–194

Cooper JE (1988) The structure and presentation of contemporary psychiatric classifications with special references to ICD-9 and 10. Br J Psychiatry [Suppl 1] 152:21–28

Cross-National Collaborative Panic Study Second Phase Investigators (to be published) Drug treatment of panic disorder: comparative efficacy of alprazolam, imipramine and placebo. Br J Psychiatry

Crow TJ (1980) Positive and negative schizophrenic symptoms and the role of dopamine. Br J Psychiatry 137:383–386

Csernansky JG, Kaplan J, Hollister LE (1985) Problems in classification of schizophrenics as neuroleptic responders and nonresponders. J Nerv Ment Dis 173:325–330

Davidson J, Pelton S (1986) Forms of atypical depression and their response to antidepressant drugs. Psychiatry Res 17:87–95

DeLisi LE, Crow TJ, Hirsch SR (1986) The Third Biannual Winter Workshop on Schizophrenia. Arch Gen Psychiatry 43:706–711

Di Nardo PA, Barlow DH, Cerny J, Vermilyea BB, Vermilyea JA, Himadi W, Waddell M (1985) Anxiety disorders interview schedule – revised (ADIS-R), phobia and anxiety disorders clinic. State University of New York at Albany, Albany, NY

Endicott J, Spitzer RL (1978) A diagnostic interview: the schedule for affective disorders and schizophrenia. Arch Gen Psychiatry 35:837–844

Feighner JP, Robins E, Guze SB, Woodruff RA, Winokur G, Munoz R (1972) Diagnostic criteria for use in psychiatric research. Arch Gen Psychiatry 26:57–63

Fenton WS, McGlashan TH, Heinssen RK (1988) A comparison of DSM-III and DSM-III-R schizophrenia. Am J Psychiatry 145:1446–1449

Fyer AJ, Mannuza S, Endicott J (1987) Differential diagnosis and assessment of anxiety: recent developments. In: HY Meltzer (ed) Psychopharmacology: the third generation of progress. Raven Press, New York

Holmberg G (1987) Anxiety disorders: classification and diagnosis. Acta Psychiatr Scand [Suppl 335] 76:7–13

Howarth BG, Grace MGA (1985) Depression, drugs, and delusions. Arch Gen Psychiatry 42:1145–1147

Joyce PR, Paykel ES (1989) Predictors of drug response in depression. Arch Gen Psychiatry 46:89–99

Klein DF, Ross DC, Cohen P (1987) Panic and avoidance in agoraphobia. Arch Gen Psychiatry 44:377–385

Liddle PF (1987) The symptoms of chronic schizophrenia. Br J Psychiatry 151:145–151

Liebowitz MR, Quitkin FM, Stewart JW, McGrath PJ, Harrison WM, Markowitz JS, Rabkin JG, Tricamo E, Goetz M, Klein DF (1988) Antidepressant specificity in atypical depression. Arch Gen Psychiatry 45:129–137

Maier W, Heuser I, Philipp M, Schlegel S, Benkert O (1988a) Diagnostic determinants of short-term spontaneous course of major depression. Psychiatry Res 23:117–118

Maier W, Philipp M, Buller R (1988b) The value of structured clinical interviews (Letter to the Editor). Arch Gen Psychiatry 45:963–964

Maier W, Heuser I, Philipp M, Schlegel S, Buller R, Wiedemann K, Benkert O (1989) The predictive ability of subtypes of depressive disorder for response to antidepressant treatment. Psychiatry Res (in press)

Moscarelli M, Maffei C, Cesana BM, Boato P, Farma T, Grilli A, Lingiardi V, Cazullo CL (1987) An international perspective on assessment of negative and positive symptoms in schizophrenia. Am J Psychiatry 144:1595–1598

Murphy DL, Shiling DJ, Murray RM (1978) Psychoactive drug responder subgroups: possible contributions to psychiatric classification. In: Lipton MA, DiMascio, Killam KF (eds) Psychopharmacology: a generation of progress. Raven Press, New York

Noyes R (1987) Drug treatment of anxiety disorders: update 1987. J Affective Dis 13:95–98

Parker G, Blignault I, Manicavasagar V (1988) Neurotic depression: delineation of symptom profiles and their relation to outcome. Br J Psychiatry 152:15–23

Paykel ES, Hollyman JA, Freeling P, Sedgwick P (1988) Predictors of therapeutic benefit from amitriptyline in mild depression: a general practice placebo-controlled trial. J Affective Dis 14:83–95

Philipp M, Maier W (1986) The polydiagnostic interview: a structured interview for polydiagnostic classification of psychiatric patients. Psychopathology 19:175–185

Philipp M, Maier W (1988) Psychopathologische Prädiktion des ambulanten Doxepin-Response. Der Nervenarzt 59:482–487

Prien RF, Kupfer DJ (1986) Continuation drug therapy for major depressive episodes: How Long Should It Be Maintained? Am J Psychiatry 143:18–23

Prusoff BA, Weissman MM, Klerman GL, Rounsaville BJ (1980) Research diagnostic criteria subtypes of depression. Arch Gen Psychiatry 37:796–801
Quitkin FM, Stewart JW, McGrath PJ, Liebowitz MR, Harrison WM, Tricamo E, Klein DF, Rabkin JG, Markowitz JS, Wager SG (1988) Phenelzine versus imipramine in the treatment of probable depression: defining syndrome boundaries of selective MAOI responders. Am J Psychiatry 145:306–311
Robins E, Guze SB (1970) Establishment of diagnostic validity in psychiatric illness. Am J Psychiatry 126:983–987
Robins LN, Helzer JE, Croughan J, Ratcliff KS (1981) The NIMH diagnostic interview schedule: its history, characteristics, and validity. Arch Gen Psychiatry 38:381–389
Robins LN, Wing J, Helzer JE (1985) WHO-ADAMHA composite international diagnostic interview. World Health Organization, Geneva
Roose SP, Glassman AH, Walsh BT, Woodring S (1986) Tricyclic nonresponders: phenomenology and treatment. Am J Psychiatry 143:345–348
Rosenthal NE, Sack DA, Gillin JC, Lewy AJ, Goodwin FK, Davenport Y, Mueller PS, Newsome DA, Wehr TA (1984) Seasonal Affective disorder. Arch Gen Psychiatry 41:72–80
Spitzer RL, Endicott J, Robins E (1970) Research diagnostic criteria: rationale and research reliability. Arch Gen Psychiatry 35:773–785
Spitzer RL, Endicott J, Robins E (1975) Clinical criteria for psychiatric diagnosis and DSM-III. Am J Psychiatry 132:1187–1192
Spitzer RL, Fleiss JL, Endicott J (1978) Problems of classification: reliability and validity. In: Lipton MA, DiMascio A, Killam KF (eds) Psychopharmacology: a generation of progress. Raven Press, New York
Spitzer RL, Williams JBW (1983) Structured clinical interview for DSM-III (SCID). Biometrics Research Department, New York State Psychiatric Institute, New York, New York
Strauss JS (1973) Diagnostic models and the nature of psychiatric disorders. Arch Gen Psychiatry 29:445–449
Strauss JS (1975) A comprehensive approach to psychiatric diagnosis. Am J Psychiatry 132:1193–1199
Strauss JS (1986) Psychiatric diagnosis: a reconsideration based on longitudinal processes. In: Millon T, Klerman GL (eds) Contemporary directions in psychopathology. Guilford Press, New York London
Wing JK (1988) Schedules for clinical assessment in neuropsychiatry (SCAN). MRC Social Psychiatry Unit, Institute of Psychiatry, London
Wing JK, Cooper JE, Sartorius N (1974) Description and classification of psychiatric symptoms. Cambridge University Press, London
World Health Organization (1978) Mental disorders: glossary and guide to their classification in accordance with the ninth revision of the international classification of diseases. World Health Organization, Geneva

# Functional Classification and Response to Psychotropic Drugs*

O. BENKERT[1]

Psychopathologically defined diagnoses represent guidelines for the application of drugs and serve as selection criteria for the evaluation of potentially useful psychopharmacological agents. Therefore, the success of research in drug evaluation strongly depends on the conceptual frameworks of diagnostic classification and how these change. For instance, at the beginning of the era of antidepressants 30 years ago, the efficacy of antidepressants was thought to be restricted to patients with endogenous depression, but since then their therapeutic spectrum has broadened: first to the "depressive syndrome" and then, due to the growing acceptance of DSM-III, to the major depressive episode. Now, even further indications for antidepressants, especially for panic disorder and generalized anxiety disorder, have been suggested.

The empirical support for the discrimination between different classes of psychotropic drugs is weak. This difficulty becomes evident in the differentiation between antidepressive and anxiolytic drugs which presupposes a psychopathological distinction between depression and anxiety. Empirical research in psychopathology, however, has not been able to establish a clear distinction between these two syndromes; in particular, the discrimination between depression and generalized anxiety has not been clearly substantiated (Angst and Dobler-Mikola 1985). Because of adherence to the postulate that depression and anxiety are clinically discriminable antidepressants were not tested as treatment for generalized anxiety. Only recently have several studies addressed this question, finding tricyclic antidepressants to be effective in treating generalized anxiety, too (McNair and Kahn 1981; Lipman et al. 1986; Kahn et al. 1986). This result argues against a sharp distinction between antidepressant and anxiolytic drugs.

But the category "anxiolytic drugs" also came to be questioned. After the distinction between panic and phobic and generalized anxiety disorder became familiar, the diagnostic category of anxiety disorder (neurosis) was considered to be of only limited validity. Klein (1964) postulated very early that imipramine specifically blocked spontaneous panic attacks. Thus, drug trials in anxiety syndromes presently are focusing on each of the three anxiety disorders sepa-

* Dedicated to Professor Dr. Hanns Hippius on the occasion of his 65th birthday.

[1] Psychiatrische Klinik der Universität Mainz, Untere Zahlbacher Straße 8, 6500 Mainz, FRG

Methodology of the Evaluation of Psychotropic Drugs
Editors: O. Benkert, W. Maier, and K. Rickels
(Psychopharmacology Series 8)
© Springer-Verlag Berlin Heidelberg 1990

rately. It could be observed that some frequently used benzodiazepines are not effective in each of the three distinct anxiety disorders: e.g., diazepam turned out to be ineffective in panic disorder although this drug is effective in generalized anxiety disorder (Shader et al. 1982; Sheehan 1982). This observation proposes a discrimination between antipanic drugs and drugs for treating generalized anxiety. However, these observations are at variance with the findings of Tyrer et al. (1988), who are calling into question the specific effect of antidepressants, benzodiazepines (and of psychological treatment strategies) in generalized anxiety, panic disorder, and dysthymic disorder: 210 outpatients with all kinds of "neurotic" disorders were randomized to placebo, dothiepin, diazepam, cognitive behavior therapy, and self-help therapy. There were no important differences in treatment response between the diagnostic groups. Consequently the term "anxiolytic" drug is misleading and may perhaps prevent an optimal treatment of patients with anxiety disorders.

Further trials have been successful in finding new *subtypes* of depression according the response to antidepressants in psychotic depression (Spiker et al. 1985), and to MAO inhibitors in atypical depression (Liebowitz et al. 1984); chronic depression is now described as dysthymia (Koscis and Frances 1987; Weissmann et al. 1988) and has been validated in pharmacotherapeutical studies (Scott et al. 1988). An attempt has been made to distinguish between severe, moderate, and mild depression by drug response studies (Paykel et al. 1988). Furthermore, the indication of high-potency serotonin re-uptake blockers such as chlorimipramine, fluoxetine, and fluvoxamin was shown to be effective in obsessive-compulsive disorder (Thoren et al. 1980; Turner et al. 1985; Perse et al. 1987). The efficacy of tricyclic antidepressants in eating disorders has been studied, too (Pope et al. 1985; Swift et al. 1986).

Although several new depressive subtypes have already been described, further subcategorization studies are in progress (Cassano et al. 1988). The multiaxial concept of DSM-III/DSM-III-R and the concept of comorbidity gives manifold possibilities to find out new correlations between psychopathological symptoms; this provides a basis to describe new subtypes, which have to be validated by psychotropic drugs. As an example let us consider the subtyping of panic disorder.

The validity of subtyping panic disorder into concurrent avoidance behavior and concurrent (secondary) major depression (MDE) was tested using the data from the Cross National Panic Study (CNPS) in c. 1100 patients; avoidance behavior and MDE were associated with an increased severity of psychopathology and a higher frequency of other DSM-III disorders at baseline; the influences of both diagnostic variables were additive or superadditive. Avoidance behavior, especially the discrimination between agoraphobic and nonagoraphobic patients, but not MDE, predicted an unfavorable response in the 8-week drug trial, independent of the particular treatment (imipramine, alprazolam, placebo). Neither avoidance behavior nor MDE are useful predictors for choosing between imipramine and alprazolam in order to optimize the treatment response (Maier et al. 1990). However, the presence of agoraphobia predicted a more unfavorable course when treated with placebo, thus indicating the special need for active treatment in panic disorder with agoraphobia. The subtyping of panic disorder is therefore useful for planning treatment.

The results about specificity or unspecificity of psychotropic drugs in subtypes should stimulate strategies for systematic investigation of the efficacy of psychotropic drugs beyond the diagnostic categories for which they are originally intended. Psychotropic drugs demonstrating antidepressive, anxiolytic, or antipsychotic efficacy in preclinical trials should be tested in the whole range of major and minor psychoses. Carefully designed assessment instruments of a broader syndrome of psychopathology and classification should be administered. Controlled clinical trials should therefore be performed in large trial groups including several diagnostic categories (e.g., depression and anxiety disorders or, depression, dysthymia, and negative schizophrenia); the scope of the trial group should be large enough to test diagnostic distinctions (e.g., between affective disorders and negative schizophrenia) for their predictive power for treatment outcome. This procedure also enables us to define the range of efficacy of psychotropic drugs in psychopathological terms independently of diagnostic conventions; the utility of classification schedules can be tested in this way. The treatment of syndromes which cannot be treated effectively up to now (e.g., negative schizophrenia) may significantly improve in this way.

It seems to be reasonable not only to look for valid subtypes but also to look for broader new valid *syndromes*. For example, it has been demonstrated that tricyclic antidepressants have an acceptable efficacy in the treatment of several subtypes of depressive disorders: panic disorder, generalized anxiety, phobic disorders, dysthymia, hyposomnia, pain, and various psychosomatic disorders. The range of efficacy of tricyclics may indicate a unitary classification for tricyclic responsive syndromes; as a preliminary proposal we will call this broad syndrome of mild to moderate severity "*minor psychiatric disorder.*" We are presently trying to determine the validity of this proposed concept in an outpatient study.

The areas of indication for antipsychotic drugs are changing too. Neuroleptics, especially atypical and new neuroleptic drugs, have to be evaluated not only on the basis of whether they are globally effective in schizophrenia but whether they demonstrate a specific efficacy for positive or negative schizophrenia or subgroups like "borderline syndromes" (Goldberg et al. 1986; Soloff et al. 1986; Cowdry and Gardner 1988). Moreover, some tricyclic neuroleptics (Robertson and Trimble 1982; Pöldinger and Sieberns 1983) or the benzamides (Benkert and Holsboer 1984) might work as antidepressants when given in low dosages. Furthermore, benzodiazepines are not only accepted anxiolytics; there is evidence that certain forms of stupor and catatonic syndromes may be effectively treated with lorazepam (Wetzel et al. 1987). Lithium and carbamazepine may prove not only to be efficient treatments in the prophylaxis of affective psychoses but seem to be effective in other episodic disorders, too (Frost and Messika 1983; Evans and Gualtieri 1985). Calcium antagonists are currently being tested for their efficacy in regard to the hypothesis that the physiological principle of "arousal" defines the target syndrome; consequently, calcium antagonists have been tested in manic syndromes (Aldenhoff et al. 1990) and in withdrawal syndromes due to alcohol abuse (Koppi et al. 1987) across the diagnostic boundaries known so far. Furthermore, several reports on the antipsychotic effect of different psychotropic drugs like propranolol, clonidine, naloxone, opioid peptides, cholecystokinin peptides, or benzodiazepines in high dosages have been published (Hollister 1987).

In summary, we have to break through psychopathologically defined boundaries. It is evident from these examples that the range of efficacy of our psychotropic drugs cannot really be described in terms of merely psychopathologically defined diagnoses according to DSM-III/DSM-III-R or RDC, which are most frequently used in drug evaluation studies. Unfortunately, there is no practicable alternative – at least not yet. It should be kept in mind that clinical diagnoses are to be considered as conventions mainly supported by the acceptance they receive from clinicians, and have been validated only by a small body of empirical data. They are also far from being perfect from a purely psychopathological point of view. The deficiency in reliability, validity, and specificity of the diagnosis of schizophrenia, for example, has been discussed thoroughly by Helmchen (1988). Consequently, modern operationalized versions of diagnostic discriminations should be considered as hypotheses (Klerman 1983) requiring empirical substantiation in the future.

Psychopathological concepts ignoring clearly defined diagnostic boundaries are not in contradiction to empirical psychopathological data. The concepts of unitary psychosis ("Einheitspsychose"; Griesinger 1867) or continuum models (Angst et al. 1983; Crow 1986) may illustrate this notion. From this point of view there is little sense in considering diagnostic categories as a sound and unquestionable basis for biological research and for clinical psychopharmacology. On the other hand, up to now the only economical and practical manner for characterizing treatment response to psychotropic drugs has been based on psychopathological features of patients being treated with these drugs. However, there is no reason to believe that a diagnostic schedule mainly based on a committee agreement could be an optimal tool for the definition of samples for treatment studies and the characterization of treatment response.

A classification of psychiatric conditions that is relevant and useful for clinical psychopharmacology should be able to identify groups of patients defined by their response to particular psychotropic drugs. Psychiatric conditions which are responsive to imipramine or other tricyclic antidepressants must be differentiated from conditions which are not responsive to these drugs; likewise, psychiatric conditions responsive to particular benzodiazepine, neuroleptic drugs, anticonvulsive drugs, or lithium should be identifiable. Psychopathological, biological, or psychosocial features predictive of drug response may be used for defining the subgroups responsive to particular drugs. Combinations of these features are being used to describe the range of efficacy of particular drugs. It is essential for these defining variables to be predictive of response to particular psychotropic drugs. This kind of classification may be called *functional classification*. The intention of functional classification is not to indicate etiologically defined nosological entities but to provide a solid basis for predicting drug response and conducting drug trials. Examples for this procedure come mainly from studies with tricyclic antidepressants where efficacy has been determined in a series of subtypes of affective disorders. Functionality refers mainly to the ability of the classification to predict treatment response to psychotropic drugs (or other sorts of therapy), being an optimal way to show the relevance of such a new approach to classification. However, an even broader interpretation of functionality in psychiatry can help to overcome premature conclusions on the specificity of drugs in the treatment of various conditions.

Thus it becomes obvious to introduce other functional aspects, such as the prediction of course or outcome, biological and possibly personality variables, and sociodemographic and social data, as well. The functional classification of psychiatric syndromes and conditions utilizes multiple levels and provides a flexible and comprehensive approach. It makes use of classification systems and subtypes proposed in the literature in a more appropriate manner. The functional classification approach helps to avoid early diagnostic and therapeutic fixations.

The functional classification is open (in the direction of a syndrome *and* subtype concept) and not tied to psychopathological conventions. The functional classification can include – as soon as they have been defined – nosological entities. The dimensional principle should be favoured, but the categorical should not be excluded. A heuristic way to introduce functional classification would be an approach applying a polydiagnostic interview flexible enough to be supplemented by new classification systems (Philipp and Maier 1986).

Another approach by von Praag et al. (1987) not relying on nosological classification systems has been proposed recently; this alternative approach chooses another framework for the psychopathological characterization of cases and of treatment response. These authors aim at the psychopathological correlates of biological psychiatry. Instead of adhering to particular diagnostic categories, they include patients with a broad variety of diagnoses in the samples under study. The patient's psychopathological features are described by a battery of items, factors, and dimensions, and these psychopathological variables are then correlated with biological characteristics. The authors call this approach "denosologization of biological psychiatry" and give evidence of its superiority to the diagnosis-based approach in psychiatric research.

This strategy is similar to the strategy proposed by Buchsbaum and Haier (1983) aiming at the inversion of dependent and independent variables. Several biological indicators like DST, SPEM, MAO activity, REM latency, and CT ventricle size, are candidates for the "select-by-marker" strategy which is intended to replace the "select-by-diagnosis" strategy. The first step of this strategy is to go beyond the psychopathological concepts by defining the patient's response in terms of biological variables. Secondly, psychopathological variables with a high correlation with the most valid biological variables are selected; the biological and psychopathological variables selected can be tested with regard to their predictive power for treatment response. In a study conducted at the Psychiatric Department of the University of Mainz, 70 former inpatients participated in a polydiagnostic follow-up interview exactly 3 years after a first examination with the DST during an active episode of a major depressive disorder (RDC), whereby the DST-suppressor/nonsuppressor status proved to be predictive of a higher rate of full remission and relapse after a symptom-free interval; this type of long-term course is assumed to be typical in endogenous depression. It is to be concluded that the subtyping of major depression according to the DST-suppressor status reveals predictive validity with respect to the long-term course (Philipp in preparation).

In any case, the issues of classification and psychopathological description need new approaches. Characterizing the sample of patients for treatment studies exclusively by a particular category of a diagnostic schedule with limited validity does not sufficiently serve the present requirements for improving treatment. On the contrary, only by considering a functional classification system will it be possible to go beyond diagnostical boundaries and to abandon the conventional limits for psychopharmacological agents, thereby avoiding the erroneous attribution of a specific efficacy to a new drug product.

Even if we set first therapeutic priority to covering a broad spectrum of psychopathological symptoms, we have to look for reliable predictive variables all the more. In describing subtypes like delusional depression, severe, moderate, and mild depression, atypical depression, hysteroid dysphoria or panic disorder, and by proving differential response to different kinds of antidepressant treatments, we have already come along a substantial part of the way. We have to continue working along these lines because there is still no unanimous agreement on valid psychopathological or clinical predictors of antipsychotic or antidepressant treatment outcome. Criteria for indication of specific treatments should be able to predict the response to the indicated treatment. The crucial status of psychopathologically defined diagnoses for the indication of specific treatments (e.g., antidepressant drugs for depressive disorders) can only be justified if the response to the indicated treatment can be predicted. To illustrate this more clearly: empirical studies demonstrating that patients diagnosed with depression (major or endogenous depression) respond more favorably to antidepressants than to neuroleptics are not available; likewise, there is no convincing evidence that all patients diagnosed with schizophrenia respond less favorably to antidepressants than to neuroleptics or to antidepressants.

In order to overcome this problem, studies randomly assigning neuroleptics and antidepressants to patients with affective and psychotic disorders seem to be necessary. Unfortunately this kind of study raises ethical concerns. For affective and schizophrenic disorders treatments are available which are considered to be efficacious, therefore, say some, the application of drugs with questionable efficacy needs ethical justification. However, this kind of study would be able to detect subtypes of disorders which may respond more favorably to certain drugs which have not been indicated for them up to now, e.g., antidepressant drugs may be more effective in treating negative schizophrenia than neuroleptic drugs. A recent study of this kind has been published by Johnstone et al. (1988). They compared the effect of the antipsychotic pimozide, lithium, and a combination of these two treatments with placebo in a 4-week trial in 120 psychotic patients with manic symptoms, depressive symptoms, and psychotic symptoms. Unfortunately, the results cannot be interpreted because of the small group of patients and a too short trial period, as well as other methodological problems (Goodwin et al. 1985).

To return to the need for functional classification: the rating scales available for the assessments of anxiety and depression for other psychiatric disorders do not fulfill the necessary conditions for measurement of treatment response. The flaws of the traditional rating scales require alternative methods for measuring the severity of the illness. Monitoring methods for behavior and autonomic function are already being tested for speech behavior, motor activity, and communicative behaviors; monitoring systems for heart rate and respiration in anxiety disorders have already been systematically developed (Taylor et al. 1986). All these measures have the advantage of being independent of observer and patient judgement. The utility of these methods for measuring the severity of symptoms and of treatment response has not yet been verified. But even if these methods turn out to be valid, they are only tapping some aspects of psychopathology, course of illness, or treatment response. Therefore, rating scales are still needed. In addition to rating scales and biological parameters, entirely different outcome criteria could be taken into consideration, such as assessment of quality of life, social and family functioning, etc. It has been demonstrated that patients with schizophrenia (Strauss and Carpenter 1974; Maj 1985) and depression (DiMascio et al. 1979; Giller et al. 1988) in treatment improve in some areas while they remain impaired in others.

The functional classification as described in this contribution recommends the inclusion of a broad range of patients and the use of a broad variety of assessment instruments in order to identify predictors of response to particular drugs. This approach promises to provide valid information on the range of efficacy and predictors of response to treatment in an economical and fast manner. The functional classification is a new conceptional approach. Of course, it must first be verified in the course of a gradual transition from the present trial methodology to the one proposed here that the functional classification concept for the evaluation of psychotropic drugs and the planning of treatment is superior to the previous procedure of strict adherence to acknowledged disease classifications.

## References

Aldenhoff JB, Schlegel S, Benkert O (1989) Gallopamil influences the manic syndrome by reducing excitement. (submitted)

Angst H, Scharfetter C, Stassen HH (1983) Classification of schizo-affective patients by multidimensional scaling and cluster analyses. Psychopathology 16:254–264

Angst J, Dobler-Mikola A (1985) The Zürich Study. VI. A continuum from depression to anxiety disorders. Eur Arch Psychiatry Neurol Sci 235:179–186

Benkert O, Holsboer F (1984) Effect of sulpiride in endogenous depression. In: Sedvall G (ed) The use of substituted benzamides in psychiatry. Acta Psychiatr Scand [Suppl 311] 39:43–48

Buchsbaum MS, Haier RJ (1983) Psychopathology: biological approaches. Annu Rev Psychol 34:401–430

Cassano GB, Musetti L, Perugi G, Soriani A, Mignani V, McNair DM, Akiskal HS (1988) A proposed new approach to the clinical subclassification of depressive illness. Pharmacopsychiatry 21:19–23

Crow TJ (1986) The continuum of psychosis and its implication for the structure of the gene. Br J Psychiatry 149:419–429

# Appendix

# National and International Guidelines for the Conduct of Clinical Trials of Psychotropic Drugs

B. MÜLLER-OERLINGHAUSEN[1]

## 1 Introduction

In the following, the essentials of existing guidelines on the performance of psychotropic and particularly antidepressant drug trials will be outlined. Belonging to this self-perpetuating community of so-called experts, whose fate is to spend hundreds of hours in national and international committees in developing various kinds of "guidelines", one often wonders, whether there is really any practical impact of all these activities. It strikes me that even colleagues, who have been working on similar documents for years, seem much inclined to forget about so much existing printed material and restart the discussion from the zero point every time.[2]

## 2 Regulatory Notes for Guidance Vs Guidelines

Before entering into the content of existing specific guidelines, the difference between guidelines and regulations must be explained. Whereas guidelines are documents of a scientific consensus, regulations present legal requirements how to perform drug trials mostly on a national level, but nowadays also on an international or European level, as can be seen from the recent drafts of general and specific guidelines and recommendations of the EEC (e.g., see the fourth draft on "Good clinical practice for trials on medicinal products in the European community" by the Committee on Proprietary Medicine and Products.)

To my knowledge, an exhaustive survey of various national requirements for clinical drug testing has never been published. However, most people would probably agree with the definition of Scoville and Crout (1978) that the main objectives of regulation can be considered to be:

[1] Department of Psychiatry, Laboratory of Clinical Psychopharmacology, Free University of Berlin, Eschenallee 3, 1000 Berlin 19, FRG

[2] For example, it seems noteworthy that even in the very scholarly chapter by J. Levine and T. Ban on "Assessment methods in clinical trials" published in *Psychopharmacology. The Third Generation of Progress* (Meltzer 1987), no international or national specific guidelines are mentioned among 117 references, although the authors refer in a very fair and differentiated way to various assessment instruments of different national origin, such as those coming from France, Italy, Germany, or Sweden.

Methodology of the Evaluation of Psychotropic Drugs
Editors: O. Benkert, W. Maier, and K. Rickels
(Psychopharmacology Series 8)
© Springer-Verlag Berlin Heidelberg 1990

1. To minimize risk to investigational subjects.
2. To assure the ethical conduct of trials.
3. To promote optimal characterization of new drugs.

"The means of accomplishing these objectives vary from country to country, although the common theme is the submission of documents to one or more authorities for review."

The situation in the U.S. is a rather specific one due particularly to the IND (Notice of Claimed Investigational Exemption for a New Drug) procedure. In contrast to countries, such as the Federal Republic of Germany or Switzerland, in the U.S. the FDA is not only responsible for the approval of a new drug application (NDA), but it also supervises and regulates all stages of the testing of a new investigational drug, thereby enforcing a very close cooperation between the sponsor, the clinical investigator, and the agency at a very early stage of drug development. Such explicit requirements for submission of documents to a central review agency before begin of a clinical trial exist also in the U.K. and in Sweden. Leber (1987) has expressed a very positive view on the IND procedure claiming that "the IND review process allows all the division's regulatory disciplines to interact in an innovative and constructive manner with those regulated, be they commercial developers, clinical investigators, or wet-bench moleculars biologists. . . . . In a way," he continues, "the IND is both a training ground and a proving ground." It seems, however, regrettable that the various national drug regulatory processes have been set up and are operating in a very autistic way without any, or only minimal reference to the procedures in other countries. To quote again from Scoville and Crout (1978): "Like pre-Bismarckian Germany, international drug testing is a maze of local and Federal interests, customs, regulations, and laws. This is, all the more apparent because of a growing international scientific consensus on how drugs should be developed, manufactured, and tested." It should be pointed out that this statement was made already 10 years ago.

In the Federal Republic of Germany, a country with one of the largest and most confusing drug markets, a new drug regulation became effective in 1978 according to which a draft of the so-called "Arzneimittel-Prüfrichtlinie" (to be translated as guidance or directive for the testing of drugs; Schnieders and Mecklenburg 1987) has been forwarded recently and will be approved in the near future. The "Arzneimittel-Prüfrichtlinie" is not a guideline in its strict sense, but it will possess legal regulatory power, and should direct the evaluation of the body of documents presented for the approval of a new drug. Indirectly it could also influence the way drugs are and will be tested in the F.R.G. and neighboring countries. On the other hand, there is a strong tendency towards the development of a practicable European drug approval process, and for many years the Federal Health Office in Berlin has based the evaluation of the documents for a new drug's approval mainly on Directive 75/318 of the EEC. The draft of the "Arzneimittel-Prüfrichtlinie," however, is not specific in any way concerning the testing of psychotropics. The same holds true for "Notification of principles for the proper execution of clinical trials on drugs" of the F.R.G. (Bundesanzeiger

1987). Its formulations and proposals are strongly influenced by the GMDS (Gesellschaft für Medizinische Dokumentation und Statistik), a politically quite powerful group of West German medical statisticians and biometricians. Also the FDA has recently forwarded a draft (May 1988) of a "Guideline for the format and content of the clinical and statistical sections of an application." This kind of "guidelines" are "intended to assist an applicant in presenting the clinical and statistical data required as part of an application under 21 CFR 314.50." Although, in most regulatory documents it is always emphasized that this "guideline describes one way, but not the only way of satisfying regulatory requirements," it can be expected that applicants will follow these instructions very carefully, taking them in fact as requirements and not just as recommendations.

## 3 Guidelines

In comparison, guidelines in the strictest sense have no direct legal impact, but they are recommendations suggesting how to perform sound clinical trials. To quote from the introductory chapter of the recently drafted new WHO consensus document "Clinical evaluation of drugs for psychiatric disorders. Principles and proposed guidelines" (version July 1987): "The main purpose of this document is education, not regulation. The recommended principles should help investigators to carry out safe and efficient evaluations. They do not include or define the regulatory or legal requirements. The described principles reflect scientific points of view of general validity" (WHO 1987).

I should add another important aspect, namely that the message of guidelines usually is directed to the less experienced investigator. Rarely do they answer the specific methodological questions of specialists.

Guidelines are usually published either by accepted public institutions, such as the WHO or the NIMH, or by ad hoc committees, or individual authors, such as a recently drafted chapter by R.F. Prien and J. Levine from the NIMH on "Research and methodological issues for evaluating the therapeutic effectiveness of antidepressant drugs."

Guidelines may refer to one or various of the following aspects:

Clinical drug trials per se
Specified phases of clinical drug testing
Testing of specified pharmacological groups
Special problems, such as drug testing in children or the elderly, transcultural problems, etc.

Also the impact of various guidelines differs markedly:

They may possess national or international relevance, or they may primarily be intended to be used in less developed countries.
The formulations of guidelines might or might not be legally required.

In the following, a short description of the various existing guidelines will be given.

## 3.1 Specific International Guidelines

Possibly the best-known example of international guidelines in the area of psychotropic drug testing are the so-called "Wittenborn" guidelines, or more formally "Guidelines for clinical trials of psychotropic drugs" (Wittenborn 1977). They were created by an ad hoc committee, which started its work in 1974 under the chairmanship of Prof. Wittenborn. The aim of this international and independent group, who worked without being influenced by any regulatory agency, pharmaceutical house, or any national scientific society, was to develop an internationally acceptable document taking as a starting point a provisional draft of the U.S. guidelines, which had been presented by the FDA at that time.

A further set of specifically international guidelines were published by the regional office for Europe of the WHO (Copenhagen) between 1983 and 1985. They are part of the European Drug Guideline Series and include separate volumes on the clinical investigation of

- Anxiolytic drugs (1983)
- Hypnotic drugs (1983)
- Antidepressant drugs (1984)
- Neuroleptic drugs (1985).

Although in many aspects they reflect the statements of the Wittenborn guidelines, they also differ from them insofar as literature references and the constituents of the special working group for each class of psychotropics is mentioned.

The working group for antidepressant drugs claims that it has consulted with experts, with the WHO member states, and with the pharmaceutical industry in order to achieve the broadest possible consensus. It is emphasized, however, that this consultation has largely been in the European region, and that these guidelines are intended to be used in the European countries. It should be added that the text has drawn also upon guidelines from two regulatory agencies, namely those of the FDA and those of the Ministry of Health of the U.S.S.R.

Hopefully in the near future, a third international document by WHO (Geneva) will be available: "Clinical evaluation of drugs for psychiatric disorders. Principles and proposed guidelines." The work on these guidelines was started in 1985 with a small working group including the president (1987) of the ECNP (European College of Neuropsychopharmacology), and also two members of the AGNP (Arbeitsgemeinschaft für Neuropsychopharmakologie und Pharmakopsychiatrie; psychopharmacological association of the German-speaking countries). Thus, the European point of view has certainly found its way also into this document. It has eight chapters, which – in contrast to the Wittenborn guidelines – do not refer to specified pharmacological groups, but to the generally accepted four phases of clinical drug testing and to special problems, such as drug testing in children, and ethical and transcultural aspects. It is the first international document in this area to explicitly cover special problems of phase 4 trials, including drug utilization studies.

## 3.2 Specific National Guidelines

The best known national guidelines are the FDA guidelines dating back to 1976 and being specified for different drug groups, such as antidepressants, hypnotics, anticonvulsants, but also to special situations, such as testing of psychoactive drugs in infants and children – the latter being a very long and comprehensive document. The existence of specific Russian guidelines was already mentioned. For the F.R.G., an updated and adapted German version of the Wittenborn guidelines was presented in a publication series of the Federal Health Office (B. Müller-Oerlinghausen and W.M. Herrmann 1981).

## 3.3 Comparison of Specific Statements from Various Guidelines

At present, there seems to exist an increased interest in holding consensus conferences and symposia on European standards of psychotropic drug testing (see Angst et al. 1989). It is said that one motive for this new enthusiasm for European standards stems from the fact that clinical investigators in Europe often feel restricted and suppressed by the strong impact of the U.S. guidelines also on trials conducted by international manufacturers in Europe. As mentioned in the introduction, however, one feels often surprised by the ignorance of some European investigators with regard what can be found in international and definitely *European* guidelines. Therefore, it might be of some interest to compare the statements of various guidelines with each other concerning well-known problems or controversies in the conduct of psychotropic drug trials. The problems of placebo control and of inclusion criteria in anti-depressant drug trials may serve as an example.

### 3.3.1 Placebo Control

Referring to the main therapeutic studies, the new WHO (Geneva) document reads as follows: "In situations where the condition may well respond to non-specific factors, such as in anxiety or in minor depressive disorder, the control should include a placebo condition." Referring to early therapeutic studies, it reads: "In severely depressed patients, only short wash-out periods can be performed, usually not longer than one week."

In the chapter on ethics, the significance of local ethic committees is stressed. On the other hand, it is pointed out that in setting up such committees, "there should be wide representation from constituencies, which may have different interests and concerns in the clinical evaluations. It has been found helpful to insure participation of representatives of psychiatrists, psychologists, nurses, and other allied professions as well as patients, their relatives, and other lay-volunteers."

The FDA guidelines on antidepressant drug trials (1977), which "have been developed largely, or entirely, by the FDA's Advisory Committees and consultants," express the following view: "In conditions, such as depression and anxiety states the superiority of standard existing drugs over placebo is of sufficiently modest extent to make the administration of placebo to some patients in a study entirely justifiable, particularly if there are explicit provisions of removing from the study patients whose clinical conditions worsen or fail to improve in a reasonable period of time."

Concerning drug-free periods, the FDA guidelines make this statement: "When safe and feasible, each study subject should have a drug-free period for several days. The number of days depend on the prior medication . . . and its duration." The FDA guidelines emphasize two reasons for this procedure: To detect and eliminate from the study rapid remitters and placebo responders, and to detect possible withdrawal symptoms of a foregoing medication. Regarding placebo or standard drug as controls in phase 2 trials, it is emphasized that "comparisons between two active drugs usually require much larger sample sizes than active drug-placebo comparisons." Concerning phase 3, it is postulated that "there is wide agreement that a number (preferably 3–5) of studies in phase 3 should compare the new compound with a placebo and with an established drug of demonstrated efficacy."

In contrast to the FDA document, the Wittenborn guidelines (1977) deal very extensively with ethical problems. The ethical question is clearly formulated: "Is it better to treat innumerable patients with a marked, but inadequately tested substance not known to be more effective than an inert placebo or . . . is it better to make deliberate investigational use of inert medication in a limited number of patients requiring treatment? . . . Although specific circumstances or prevailing ethics may contraindicate the use of placebo comparisons, claims for efficacy must provide an acceptable alternative, e.g. comparisons of dosage response curve." (Later on it is specified that at least two different doses should be examined; another alternative would be a design where a group receiving the investigational drug is compared with a group receiving placebo in terms of the amount of standard supplementation required to maintain patients at some specific levels.) The chapter continues: "In psychopharmacology, masses of data are not regarded as an acceptable alternative for studies involving unambiguous comparisons."

Quoting the passages of the FDA document mentioned before, the Wittenborn guidelines point out that in some countries the ethics of the use of placebo, especially in depressed outpatients, is questioned. However, they also emphasize that many investigators would principally question the use of suicidal patients in drug trials regardless of whether placebo control is involved or not.

The WHO Europe guidelines are mostly in line with the recommendations of the other guidelines quoted so far. They suggest that the very early trials should be performed only in hospitalized patients, excluding severely depressed and potentially suicidal patients altogether during phase 2 trials. They also ask for a number of placebo-controlled studies. The ethical problem of use of placebo appears not to be seen primarily under the aspect of prolonged suffering of a severely depressed patient, but under the aspect of the risk of suicide. The document says that studies which may involve such risks should only be conducted if the patient is adequately safeguarded and the procedure is considered to be ethically justified.

In summary, all existing guidelines seem to agree upon the principal benefit and the feasibility of placebo-controlled trials in depressed patients.

### 3.3.2 Selection of Patients for Antidepressant Drug Trials

An often discussed point of controversy refers to the sample characteristics of patients for antidepressant drug trials ("homogeneity" or "heterogeneity"?). The WHO Europe guidelines suggest choosing very heterogeneous samples in early phase 2, and samples as homogeneous as possible in late phase 2 studies. Most guidelines recommend the inclusion of outpatients in late phase 2 and phase 3 trials.

Concerning the classification and description of trial patients, the Wittenborn and FDA guidelines do not recommend specific classification systems. However, they stress the point that regardless which classification criteria are used, patients should also be carefully described in terms of socio-demographic and clinical characteristics. Only the WHO Europe guidelines specify available classification systems, such as ICD, RDC, DSM-III, CATEGO, Vienna Research Criteria. They also emphasize that the investigator would be well advised to use an internationally recognized method with which he has had successful personal experience and training.

The WHO Europe and the Wittenborn guidelines unanimously agree on the assumption that antidepressant drug treatment may be useful not only for depression as a "syndrome," but also for depression as a "symptom." However, they also emphasize that patients admitted to a study on the treatment of depression as a "symptom," should be carefully characterized and quantified in all respects since it is not clear that a drug effective in one type of such depression will necessarily be effective in another. The WHO Europe guidelines clearly state that patients with only mild changes of mood can hardly be considered as pathologically depressive and are not suitable subjects for "studies involving new drugs."

## 3.4 Conclusion

In conclusion, as the most economical procedure it would appear that before issuing new directives or consensus documents, the experts should reflect the concurrent recommendations of the existing guidelines as a starting point and also as proof for a rather far-reaching basic international consensus in the area of drug testing including antidepressant drug trials. There seems to be much more concordance than factual discordance in these documents, although the formulations obviously are sometimes more rigid and more pressing in the FDA's than in the international guidelines. Specific methodological issues, however, such as problems of the validity and utility of specified scales to be used in specified countries, the usefulness of routinely assessed "biological markers," etc. can hardly be answered in a definite way by guidelines, which by definition should not aim at more than delineating the state of the art in a general and therefore widely acceptable way. The rest is and should be up to the results of more or less localized scientific discussion and the responsibility of experienced investigators. Documents of a more regulatory nature should not try to go beyond this imminent and plausible limit of "guidelines" in their proper sense, apart from specified directives of a purely organizational character.

## References

Angst J et al. (1989) Consensus conference on the methodology of clinical trials of antidepressants, Zürich, March 1988: report of the consensus committee. Pharmacopsychiatry 22:3-7

Bundesminister für Jugend, Familie, Frauen und Gesundheit (1987) Bekanntmachung von Grundsätzen für die ordnungsgemäße Durchführung der klinischen Prüfung von Arzneimitteln. Bundesanzeiger 243:16617 (30.12)

Leber P (1987) FDA: the federal regulation of drug development. In: Melzer HJ (ed) Psychopharmacology. The third generation of progress. Raven Press, New York

Levine J, Schiele BC, Bouthilet L (1971) Principles and problems in establishing the efficacy of psychotropic agents. Public Health Service Publication No. 2318, US Government Printing Office, Washington DC

Meltzer HJ (ed) (1987) Psychopharmacology. The third generation of progress. Raven, New York

Müller-Oerlinghausen B, Herrmann WM (eds) (1981) Anleitung zur klinischen Prüfung von Psychopharmaka. AMI-Berichte, Dietrich Reimer Verlag, Berlin

Schnieders B, Mecklenburg R (eds) (1987) Zulassung und Nachzulassung von Arzneimitteln. Aesopus Verlag, Basel, pp 256-269

Scoville B, Crout JR (1978) Regulations and clinical drug testing. In: Clark WG, del Giudice J (eds) Principles of psychopharmacology, 2nd edn. Academic Press, New York, pp 461-466

Wittenborn JR (ed) (1977) Guidelines for clinical trials of psychotropic drugs. June 1, 1977. Pharmacopsychiatry 10:205-231

# Subject Index